A SEEKER'S GUIDE TO THE YOGA SUTRAS

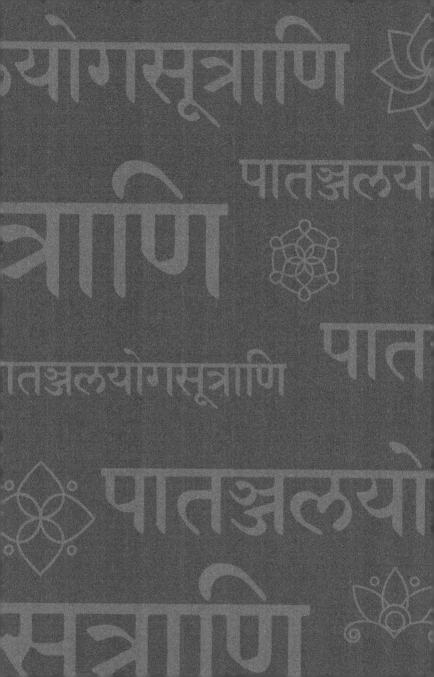

A SEEKER'S GUIDE
TO THE
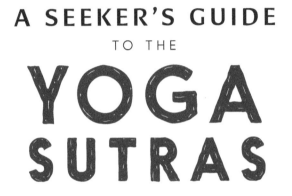
YOGA SUTRAS

MODERN REFLECTIONS
ON THE
ANCIENT JOURNEY

RAM BHAKT

ROCKRIDGE
PRESS

First Rockridge Press trade paperback edition 2019

Paperback ISBN: 978-1-64152-752-1 | ebook ISBN: 978-1-64152-753-8

Manufactured in the United States of America

Interior and Cover Designer: Tricia Jang
Art Producer: Sara Feinstein
Editor: Rochelle Torke
Production Manager: Oriana Siska
Production Editor: Melissa Edelburn

All illustrations used under license from Shutterstock.com.

Author photo courtesy of © Toph Bocchiaro

10 9 8 7 6 5 4 3 2 1

TO MY FAMILY,
FRIENDS, TEACHERS,
AND
FELLOW STUDENTS

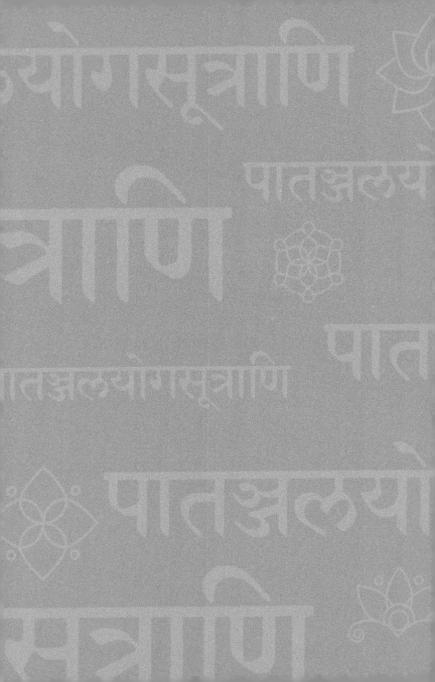

CONTENTS

Introduction **viii**

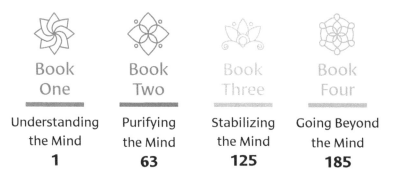

Book
One

Understanding
the Mind
1

Book
Two

Purifying
the Mind
63

Book
Three

Stabilizing
the Mind
125

Book
Four

Going Beyond
the Mind
185

Resources **212**

INTRODUCTION

I first came across *The Yoga Sutras of Patanjali* when I started training to become a yoga teacher. After reading through the sutras, and regarding the gentle face of Swami Satchidananda on the back, I felt an inner spaciousness. That inner sensation made a big impression on me. It sparked my curiosity and set me on a path to learn as much as I could about this ancient text.

This enthusiasm led me to Yogaville Ashram—a retreat founded by Swami Satchidananda in 1980. There I had the opportunity to study and live in a community devoted to the yogic lifestyle. During morning meditation sessions and in my dreams there, I started to understand the deepest parts of myself for the first time. How I reacted to events and how I treated others started to shift. I began to experience longer stretches of inner peace.

I met David Frawley in Yogaville at his training session called "Yoga and Ayurveda for Yoga Teachers." He taught us that our separation from nature and improper use of the senses creates disease and unhappiness. It was his scholarly approach and explanation of natural healing, spiritual theories, and practices that confirmed my experiences and inspired me to go to India to continue learning.

Since then, I've dedicated myself to sharing what I know and inspiring others. My childhood dream was to practice medicine. Now I promote health in a different way, spreading the message of looking within and to nature to restore our original vitality.

It is the birthright of everyone to live a life of ease, peace, and purpose. As Patanjali says, the key is discipline, study, and surrender.

This book is a practical guide to the yoga sutras of Patanjali. It is a contemporary interpretation that will help you bridge a wonderful ancient text with your modern life. It reveals the possibilities for an accelerated journey of the soul by following a dedicated practice of yoga. Unlike other translations and commentaries, I've attempted to present (in simple terms) short reflections on a selection of sutras that make them accessible to anyone.

Because yoga is an experiential science, art, and lifestyle, I encourage you to do more than contemplate the sutras. For this reason I've included a reflection, story, or a short activity to help you interact with each teaching in this book and make it your own.

I invite you to use this book however you feel it will best serve your vision for your life. You could read it front to back or dive in when you need a moment of inspiration. For deeper study, please see the Resources section (see page 212) in the back. May your exploration of this ancient and sometimes esoteric text be fruitful. Approach it with an open heart and mind and let your inner wisdom arise.

Peace and Love,

Ram Bhakt

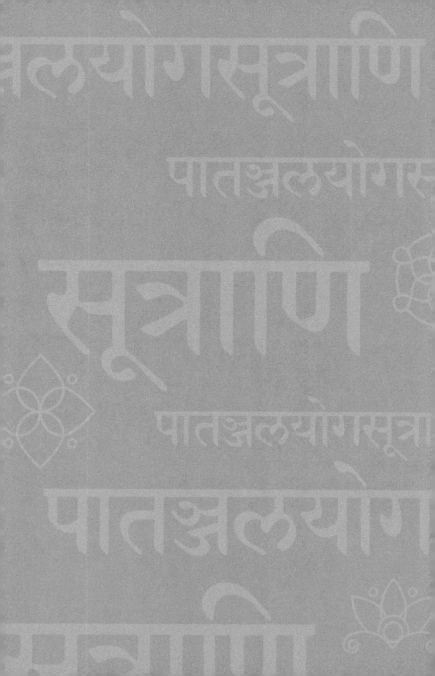

BOOK ONE

Understanding the Mind

The first book is on higher consciousness. It is about understanding and discovering our spiritual nature which is beyond the mind. Some sutras are remarkably brief, inviting us to draw them into ourselves thoughtfully, reflecting on each word.

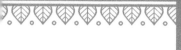

The Value of Learning

1.1 NOW YOGA IS EXPLAINED.

When you seek to know life beyond the surface level or you aspire to actively transform your experience into wisdom and growth, you are ready for yoga. This book is about how to make the mind infinitely receptive and calm—and how to transcend the mind itself.

Yogic teachings are timeless because they can reduce confusion and suffering—challenges faced by humans in all ages.

This first sutra is a simple invitation to step inside, to begin a new relationship with your mind and your identity, and to determine how you will spend your precious time here on Earth.

Others have gone before us who, out of love and compassion, have shared their experiences to help us on the path. Patanjali is one such teacher. He invites us to a form of spiritual life based on a deep exploration of the nature of reality. This yogic path encourages us to clarify our perception of ourselves by recognizing our true identity beyond the mind, body, emotions, or present circumstances.

When applied sincerely, yogic wisdom helps you manage your reactions to daily experiences—not by "fixing" others or overhauling your circumstances but by helping you live instead from your true center, which is always at peace.

EXERCISE:

Take a deep breath and be grateful to be alive, to have found this book, and to learn. Take a deep breath and feel grateful to be alive.

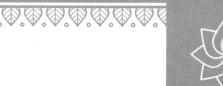

Seeing Reality Clearly

1.2 KEEPING THE MIND CALM AND FOCUSED IS THE ESSENCE OF YOGA.

Have you ever had trouble going to sleep? You want to drift off, but you are stewing over old memories or rehearsing actions you plan to take. Such thoughts and feelings come from a turbulent mind.

It is difficult for most people to keep the mind still and focused on the ideas they choose. How often does your mind stray from the present? Do you ever ask it to think about one thing but it keeps drifting to something else? Does your mind ever gather information and interpret it the wrong way? You decide a friend is ignoring you, for example, but discover later that they simply didn't get your message. Did your mind create a story that you started to believe?

The mind is a filter between you and the outside world. It can make your perception of situations better or worse. The mind is not the enemy, though; it's like an untrained animal—if it is not trained properly, it can take you for some wild rides. Be patient with it. Through the practice of yoga, you will learn how to focus the mind and make it your friend. Eventually, it will help you solve any problem or know anything without prejudice and imagination. When used properly, the mind is an incredible tool.

REFLECTION:

Think about a time when you saw a situation differently than another person. What kind of emotions or thoughts influenced your ability to see the truth?

The Higher Self

1.3 WHEN THE MIND IS CALM, THE SPIRIT EXPERIENCES ITSELF.

The real you is not your mind. Your thoughts, emotions, and body constantly move, but there is a witness within you that doesn't change—your spirit. It is the spirit that uses the mind and body to experience the outside world. There is a unique but similar spirit in everyone else, too.

The spirit is like a constant light. It has no name. It does not feel pain. It has no likes or dislikes. Right now within you, there is an exuberant spirit taking delight in watching the world. Whenever you are completely involved in what you are doing, you experience the creative and timeless nature of the spirit.

To know, connect to, and experience this inner aspect of your being is the purpose of yoga. You experience the spirit when the mind is calm. Knowledge and experience of the spirit stops overthinking and attachment. It makes you fearless and gives you more energy to play your part in life and to identify yourself not with the mind and body but with the higher self.

EXERCISE:

Take time to watch a sunset or sunrise. Allow this experience into your heart. As you do, notice how you appreciate your life and who you really are deep inside.

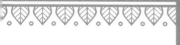

Life's Challenges

1.4 WHEN THE MIND IS MOVING, THE SPIRIT IDENTIFIES ITSELF WITH MENTAL STATES.

When you have an exuberant experience of life, you say to yourself, "Life is amazing" or "Love is everywhere." In other words, you're in a great mood. Then you have an unpleasant experience and you say, "Life is horrible." Well, which one is it? The mind is constantly making judgments and creating opinions. When you get angry, you say, "I am angry." Actually, only your mind has changed for a moment.

The fundamental you (the spirit) does not change. How you think about life challenges can make things worse than they need to be. As a yoga practitioner, every moment that you bring your mind back to the present, you start over again and renew your connection to the spirit.

Bringing the mind back to stillness or calm reminds you that mental states are only passing moments that do not touch the essence within you. The mind's own turbulence can be a powerful catalyst for spiritual growth. Doesn't a day spent with heavy or angry thoughts make you wish that much more for a deeper connection to the truth, to your own soul? Don't get angry at the disturbed mind. Thank it for also reminding you to continue your journey.

EXERCISE:
Write down every thought you have for five minutes or so. On completing this stream-of-consciousness writing, bring your attention to the part of you that has been witnessing your thoughts and life story. Who is this part of you?

Pain and Pleasure

1.5 THERE ARE FIVE TYPES OF MENTAL MODIFICATIONS, WHICH ARE EITHER PAINFUL OR PAINLESS.

As the mind shifts from one state to another, you experience pleasure or pain. The impressions left behind from these mental states affect the way that you see yourself and the world. For example, if someone gets into a car accident, they may suffer whenever they remember the painful experience even if there is no harmful event happening to them in the present.

Maybe you know people who drink alcohol or take drugs to take their mind off uncomfortable thoughts. Some people overeat or get addicted to other activities because they want to avoid certain ideas or feelings. It is possible to find yourself in a painful cycle. Through yoga practice, however, we always have the power to free ourselves from unpleasant states by learning to still the mind naturally.

Remember that both painful and pleasant experiences can lead to knowledge and realization; therefore, there's no need to race away from pain or to exhaust yourself chasing pleasures. There are lessons available in each.

REFLECTION:

Think about a time that you experienced pain. Where did it come from? Where did it go?

The Constantly Changing Mind

1.6 THE MENTAL MODIFICATIONS ARE RIGHT KNOWLEDGE, WRONG KNOWLEDGE, IMAGINATION, SLEEP, AND MEMORY.

This sutra draws our attention to the machinery of the mind—how the mind works for us on a daily basis. The mind has three functions: to know, to will, and to retain. The knowledge that you get from the world is either true or untrue depending on where you get it. When it goes into your memory, you can recall the information. Sometimes you imagine things that are not there because of previous images and thoughts. The sleep that is mentioned in this sutra is referencing the deep sleep state when you have no dreams.

By becoming aware of these states and realizing that they are passing, you can distance yourself from them and become the master of your mind. Every moment that you shine your awareness on the mind, you see how each mental state comes and goes.

There is no consistent and permanent mental state. Only the higher self, or the spirit that witnesses and observes these states, is enduring and unchanging.

REFLECTION:

Other than your knowledge, imagination, and memories, which come and go, do you experience another part of yourself that simply observes all of these states and mental activities?

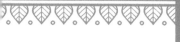

Connecting to the Truth

1.7 SOURCES OF RIGHT KNOWLEDGE ARE DIRECT PERCEPTION, INFERENCE, AND RELIABLE TESTIMONY.

The best way to know something is through direct experience. If you try something yourself, then nobody can take away what you learn or convince you of the opposite. This knowledge can be gained from personal experiences or realizations that do not require the senses, like through meditation.

The yogic sciences are founded on the universal experiences (inner or outer) of seekers throughout time. An honest and trustworthy teacher who shares from direct experience is a reliable source of knowledge. Sacred texts, like *The Yoga Sutras*, are considered true because they have withstood the test of time and have helped countless people on their path.

From past experiences and with logical thinking, you can infer or predict what might happen next. Since starting my yogic journey, I have been able to better control the outcome of my actions because I have followed the advice of my mentors. I have noticed that my senses have become sharper and that I can think more logically about situations, people, and problems in my life. Yoga makes you like a scientist who can see clearly and connect to common sense.

REFLECTION:

Think back on a positive or negative experience. What did you learn from it? Did it change your assumptions about people, situations, and problems in your life?

Living in Our Stories, Not Reality

1.8 WRONG KNOWLEDGE COMES FROM A FALSE UNDERSTANDING OF WHAT IS REAL.

Have you ever thought something was true and then found out you were wrong? It happens a lot when you assume you know something or make a generalization without firsthand experience. The senses can be especially misleading. Sometimes you hear something in the distance and think you know what it is, but you are completely wrong.

Past experiences and conditioning can blur or confuse our perception of things. If you've had a negative episode with someone, you might assume that everyone who is similar to them is to be mistrusted or avoided. This tendency for the mind to create its own assumptions and realities not only keeps us from seeing people as they are; it keeps us from seeing our own higher self as it really is.

This sutra reminds us to practice calming and centering the mind—coaxing it out of its assumed concepts and ideas.

REFLECTION:
Think about someone you don't like. Are you judging them on the basis of your beliefs, background, or experiences?

Using Your Imagination Wisely

1.9 IMAGINATION COMES FROM WORDS THAT HAVE NO CONNECTION TO REALITY.

Imagination is the third type of mental state. Unlike the first two mental modifications, right knowledge and wrong knowledge, which are concerned with the understanding of an object, imagination is completely subjective. It is a unique creation that comes from mixing words, concepts, and images into something that doesn't really exist.

In some yoga practices (like the postures), you might imagine a line of energy that is moving through the body that is invisible, but later you will feel it. When you think about possible outcomes during creative problem solving, imagining things can also be useful. At other times, however, because of feelings and desires, the mind goes through a series of thoughts that are useless, are harmful, or distort the truth. Through your yoga practice, notice that these types of thoughts diminish.

REFLECTION:

Think about a time that you anticipated a future event and created all kinds of expectations, fears, and mental drama. Did this imagining cause unnecessary suffering? Similarly, think of a time when you were lost in a reverie about something you looked forward to. Did you imagine every detail of how an exciting day in the future might unfold? Were you disappointed when things didn't turn out as expected?

The Lessons of Sleep

1.10 DREAMLESS SLEEP IS A STATE OF MIND IN WHICH THERE IS NO PERCEPTION.

During dreams, the senses are inactive but thinking continues. Images, desires, thoughts, and memories are experienced and processed by the mind. Deep sleep starts when dreams end. It occurs when you have no mental experience other than emptiness in the mind caused by a feeling of heaviness and mental inaction. It's an involuntary and unconscious state of mind.

When you wake up after a deep sleep, don't you remember not having thoughts? There is an unbroken awareness that yogis connect to that actually always exists during waking, dreaming, and the deep sleep state.

Meditation is like trying to go to sleep but staying aware at the same time. If you fall asleep while trying to meditate or feel heaviness in the mind and body, then it's best to catch up on your sleep or not eat heavy meals before meditation.

EXERCISE:

Before going to sleep tonight, write down all of your plans for the next day in a journal. Think to yourself that life itself is like a dream, and consider how you might act if you realized this.

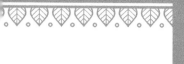

When Memories Arise

1.11 MEMORY IS HOLDING ON TO OBJECTS PERCEIVED.

Memory is made up of right knowledge, wrong knowledge, imagination, and sleep. We need memories to learn and make informed decisions, but sometimes they can be useless. What's the point of remembering something that causes you pain or that distracts you from what you are doing? During the writing of this book, memories have resurfaced and distracted me from writing. It happens to all of us.

Sometimes, because you haven't fully processed an experience or because the experience was very dramatic and you are attached to it, the memory of it keeps popping up in the back of the mind. This distraction happens especially during the early stages of meditation.

Memories recur when we consciously recall them, or they come from the unconscious part of us when we release control, like during meditation. When you slow down and create a space in the mind, memories rise to the surface and disconnect you from the present moment. Sometimes imagination distorts memory; you can have false memories or remember something incorrectly.

Although not all memories are helpful, it is important to learn from positive and negative ones equally.

REFLECTION:

What are some of your favorite memories? What are some unpleasant memories? Reflect on what they teach you about who you are and how you can use them for your growth and development.

Limitations of Sensory Pleasures

1.12 THESE FIVE MOVEMENTS OF MIND ARE CONTROLLED BY REPEATED PRACTICE AND NONATTACHMENT.

To succeed in keeping the mind calm, you must strive to understand its tendencies and to train it through practice. Every time that you bring your awareness to the present moment, you have made an effort to bring your mind and perception to order. The more you do so with yoga, the stronger and more purified your mind becomes. It starts to get into the habit of being still and clear instead of agitated or dull.

The other key is nonattachment or dispassion, which means not being caught up in expectations or sensual pleasures. Unless you have the right attitude, worldly pleasures create unhealthy cravings and attachments to things that you cannot hold on to forever and that do not bring permanent happiness.

STORY:

I spent one month in an ashram, cleaning rooms and toilets every day. I ate simple food every day. I would think about what I was doing with my life, my previous relationships, and what I was going to do when I left the ashram. After the second week, I had very vivid dreams and suddenly thereafter, I was happy for absolutely no reason. My mind had started to regain its original purity and joy from a consistent, simple, and selfless lifestyle.

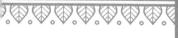

All Effort Counts

1.13 PRACTICE IS THE EFFORT TO KEEP THE MIND STILL.

There are various ways in yoga to make the mind still. My favorites are through study, physical activity, working on the breath, repeating a mantra, and helping others without expectation. People of different temperaments require different practices, but the effect is always the same—to make the mind calm and still.

For some people, the mind might already be very focused and calm. For most of us, however, if we do nothing, the mind will get into all kinds of trouble. Attached to the senses, memories, and thoughts, the mind cannot be stilled to allow the joy of the spirit to be experienced. For many, the spirit gets caught up with the mind, and the objects of pleasure and desire pull us in every direction.

What is required is a constant awareness that you are actually not the mind or the body, but you are the spirit that is temporarily using these instruments to have an experience. Slowly, you start to view life as if it were a movie that you are just watching from inside. It's like developing a double awareness: one of the outside world (including the mind and body) and the other of the inner you that is unchanging.

REFLECTION:

What are some things that agitate your mind? Practice thinking about these things as more of a distant observer instead of as a participant.

Consistency Is Best

1.14 PRACTICE BECOMES FIRMLY GROUNDED WHEN CARRIED OUT FOR A LONG TIME, WITHOUT ANY BREAK, AND WITH DEVOTION.

There are many temptations in the world and many habits, memories, and desires within each of us. To transform the mind, diligent practice is best. Sometimes people go on retreat for that reason—so they can spend more time practicing, getting established in a routine, and being inspired by others.

As you practice calming the mind in a more consistent way, you start to feel more inner peace. This result encourages you to keep practicing and to stay away from those things that disturb your connection to that peace.

Devotion to the practice comes from understanding that there are others who have gone before you and have been successful. Even if you cannot keep a regular practice, remember that life is also teaching you spontaneously. Practice is just what accelerates learning and realization.

STORY:
I practiced a mantra for about 40 days before bedtime. On the last day, I heard the mantra during my sleep! Suddenly I felt a deep, warm, glowing sensation in my mind and body. I woke up with a feeling of absolute awe.

Don't Cling to External Things

1.15 NONATTACHMENT IS THE STATE OF MENTAL MASTERY FREE FROM CRAVINGS FOR SENSE OBJECTS EITHER SEEN OR HEARD.

As long as you have a mind, you have desires. The best desire is to know your true self. Nonattachment takes willpower and practice. It is something that comes with time and experience. For example, after eating too many sweets or too much greasy food, you get sick or become very low in energy. In the future, you might choose not to overeat and start to understand the value of moderation.

It's not necessary to give up vices cold turkey. As long as you remain aware of the consequences of your thoughts and actions, your relationship with things will change.

Even the practice of yoga should not be colored by attachment and expectation for the results. You will hear and read in books many amazing effects from yoga practice, but you should always stay focused on where you are and not expect fireworks. Nonattachment allows you to maintain your balance and inner silence in all situations.

EXERCISE:

The next time you are offered something that you know might be bad for you, turn it down. You will notice a rush of energy from letting the attachment go.

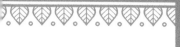

You Are Beyond All Mental States

1.16 THE HIGHEST DETACHMENT IS LACK OF ANY DESIRE FOR ANY MENTAL QUALITIES. IT COMES FROM THE EXPERIENCE OF THE SPIRIT.

There is a cyclic changing of the mind among various qualities during the day. It exists in one of three states: inertia, activity, or lightness. Inertia is when the mind feels heavy—like right before you go to bed. Activity is when the mind is alert and processing, like during midday when you are working or studying. Lightness is when the mind is very passive and clear, as might naturally occur during sunrise and sunset.

Practices like detachment, meditation, moderation, and compassion build this lightness within, but they can't completely insulate you from the stresses of the world. So the highest detachment comes when you know that you are the spirit and can observe these states of mind and not cling to any of them—even the ones that are very pleasant and light.

The experience of the spirit is always with you. Yoga allows the spiritual awareness to grow within you and become permanent—a state that doesn't fluctuate when challenges arise. With the highest level of detachment achieved, you can accomplish anything in the world and have a reserve of inner peace to support you.

EXERCISE:

The next time you are in a difficult situation, keep reminding yourself that it will pass. There is greatness within you, and the spirit is always with you!

You Become What You Focus On

1.17 COMPLETE UNDERSTANDING (*SAMPRAJNATA SAMADHI*) FOLLOWS REASONING, REFLECTION, AND THE EXPERIENCE OF BLISS AND PURE I-AM-NESS.

In this sutra, Patanjali introduces the concept of *samadhi*, which is an engrossment in your highest and truest self. It is the refinement of your inner focus and path to wisdom, the goal of yoga.

When your mind comes to a state of focus, you can understand the nature of things. During meditation, first you go into deep thought on an object or idea. You start to analyze it from every angle and go through various logical reasoning steps.

A more subtle internal state follows that is like intuition and reflection. An intelligence arises within you, and you start to know deeply the object or idea from this concentrated internal watching.

Suddenly thereafter, there is an experience of pure bliss, and then you feel like only you exist in the world! From this type of meditative experience, you come to realize how perception and knowledge arise: first comes the ego, then feeling, then subtle thoughts, and finally, concrete thoughts. Complete understanding is attained from experiencing this process.

STORY:

As a student of music, I was initially very concerned with every single note on the page. After many years of practice, the music flows without overthinking. I feel joy when I play. Now, I am a musician, not just a student.

Your Past Becomes Wisdom

1.18 THE OTHER ABSORPTION (*ASAMPRAJNATA SAMADHI*) RESULTS FROM COMPLETE CESSATION OF THE MODIFICATIONS OF THE MIND.

When you constantly practice stilling the movements of the mind with the highest detachment discussed in Sutra 1.16 (see page 32), then subconscious and unconscious materials come to the surface of the mind, and you become absorbed in them. This other type of *samadhi* (meditative absorption) is different from the one described in the previous sutra because there is no external object on which you focus the mind. Instead, the object comes from your past impressions.

From this experience, you start to empty the store of impressions in the mind from your current and previous lives! It is these deep-seated impressions (*samskaras*) that motivate you to do things and affect the way that you perceive reality.

Meditation is like going to a psychologist who asks you to talk about what has happened in your life. After talking and thinking about your past for a while, eventually the confusion, pain, or discomfort starts to lessen. Slowly, you let go of the trauma and find your inner peace again.

STORY:

During a 10-day silent meditation retreat, I suddenly remembered someone I had hurt in the past. At the same time, I realized there was nothing I could do about it and forgave myself.

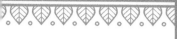

Challenges Are Steps You Climb Daily

1.30 THE DISTRACTIONS OF THE MIND ARE DISEASE, DULLNESS, DOUBT, CARELESSNESS, LAZINESS, CRAVING, FALSE PERCEPTION, FAILURE TO REACH FIRM GROUND, AND SLIPPING FROM THE GROUND GAINED. THEY ARE OBSTACLES IN YOGA.

When you are sick, your mind cannot be sharp. The last thing you want to do is meditate. All of us experience distractions and laziness at times that make steady progress difficult.

I remember many times when, after gaining deep insights and inner strength from practice, I stopped practicing. I started staying out late with friends and doing some things I shouldn't have. The next day, I would feel drained of energy, more easily distressed, and in a bad mood. I can get lazy if I do not have a set routine in my day or some goal that I am working toward. When I make practice a habit, I am always in a better mood and feel energized and enthusiastic about life.

It is not easy to practice constantly or to change habits overnight. For that reason, becoming established in a healthy yogic lifestyle and renewing your resolve daily are necessary.

REFLECTION:
What healthy resources can you use to help you get through difficult times?

Mind and Body Are Connected

1.31 THE SYMPTOMS THAT ACCOMPANY THE DISTRACTED STATE OF MIND INCLUDE PAIN, SADNESS, ANXIETY, AND IRREGULAR BREATHING.

When the mind gets distracted by the obstacles mentioned in the preceding sutra, it becomes unstable. Unstable mental patterns can affect your body because your thoughts create real forces within it. Have you ever felt discomfort in your stomach from stress? Or have you ever gotten a headache from thinking too much?

In the ancient Indian medical system called Ayurveda, there is a psychobiological force called *vata*. This force controls all the movements of the body, including the breathing process and the movement of thoughts in the mind. It is also intimately connected to the nervous system, which controls the sensation of pain.

There are diet and lifestyle recommendations for people who have more of a tendency toward imbalance of this force in them. An unhealthy body that is not supplied with good food, exercise, clean water, fresh air, and rest is unable to penetrate into the deeper aspects of the mind.

EXERCISE:

The next time you are really stressed or angry, take a moment to slow down and stabilize your breathing. Take a break and allow your mind and nervous system to regain their balance.

Sacrifice and Focus for Mastery

1.32 TO PREVENT THESE OBSTACLES AND ACCOMPANIMENTS, PRACTICE ON ONE SUBJECT.

The best way to manage your mind and nervous system is to focus on one thing at a time.

Concentrating on one thing creates a habit in your system that helps it find stability. It prevents anxiety and shallow understanding. Focused study and practice are the only way to become an expert in any subject.

When you think you can become the master of many things at once, it usually means you haven't studied what it takes. If you want to become successful in any task or project, you must prioritize that goal and sacrifice other pursuits for some time.

There was a time when I was practicing Hatha (physical) Yoga and kung fu together. I realized that each tradition has its own method of practice even though the goal might be similar in the end. To me, stretching and cultivating stillness seemed more sustainable than jump kicks and breaking objects with my hands. I chose to focus on yoga because I didn't want to practice fighting people; my goal is to become peaceful and nonviolent.

EXERCISE:

Ask someone you admire what sacrifices they made to become successful in their chosen career or path.

Four Types of People

1.33 PEACE OF MIND COMES FROM CULTIVATING AN ATTITUDE OF FRIENDLINESS TOWARD THOSE WHO ARE HAPPY, COMPASSION FOR THOSE WHO SUFFER, GOODWILL TOWARD THE VIRTUOUS, AND INDIFFERENCE TOWARD THE NONVIRTUOUS.

In the next seven sutras, Patanjali lists some specific ways to keep the mind calm and stabilize it for progress on your inner journey. Because humans are social beings, he talks about how to adjust yourself in order to deal with others. There are four types of people in his view: happy, suffering, good, or bad.

When you see a happy person, do you sometimes get jealous and wonder why they are happy and you are not? It's better to take delight in their happiness and enjoy it with them. Maybe they can teach you something.

When you see someone who is in pain, do you think you are superior to them? Or do you sometimes ignore them because they make you feel overwhelmed? Instead, it is better to respond with compassion and maybe try to help when you can.

When you see a monk or holy person, do you think they are just a dropout or being lazy? It's better to wish them success or ask for a blessing.

Lastly, do you let mean people or cheaters make you angry? Do you get caught up, analyzing and criticizing all that they're doing wrong? It's better to just ignore them and protect your inner peace.

EXERCISE:

The next time you run into someone from the nonvirtuous group, try to have minimal contact that will result in a neutral interaction.

As You Breathe, So You Think

1.34 OR THE MIND CAN BE CALMED BY EXHALING AND HOLDING THE BREATH.

The mind and the breath are intimately connected. If you pay careful attention, you notice that your breathing is irregular during moments of stress, anger, or excitement. The first thing that happens when you are scared is that you gasp for air and hold it.

Breathing is slower and smoother when you are calm and focused. It is one of the automatic processes in the body that can also be consciously controlled. If you practice watching and regulating the breath, you regulate the mind.

Always breathe through the nose and keep your abdominal muscles relaxed to get the most benefit from the breathing process. Start with lengthening the time for exhalation; do not hold the breath. After a couple of minutes of slow and deep breathing, you can try to hold the breath out for a few moments. This will calm your nerves, and anger and anxiety will go away.

EXERCISE:

Try the described breathing exercise to stabilize the mind. Notice if it is possible to have a thought when you hold the breath out.

Feeling Overrides Thinking

1.35 OR THE MIND CAN BE STEADIED
BY FOCUSING ON SUBTLE SENSE
PERCEPTIONS.

The body does its best to bring your attention to important changes in the environment. Ten seconds ago, did you feel your clothes against your skin? You probably didn't because they have been there all day and you don't need to. If you adjust your clothes, or pay really close attention, then you can feel them again. Reading this paragraph alone has drawn attention to where you feel your clothes touching your skin.

It is difficult to have a conscious thought and to feel at the same time. Focusing on very light sensations in the body, sounds, or smells helps concentrate and calm the mind. In some meditation practices, you might be asked to focus on the area of the upper lip right under the nostrils. After several days of practice, the sensations become stronger and your mind becomes easily stabilized and able to focus.

When you sit to meditate, you will start to notice very slight feelings throughout the body. Try to focus on them and watch how they change or move around. Do not immediately scratch every itch or adjust the body at the first moment of discomfort—remain detached. As you patiently wait and notice, more subtle sensations will arise, and you can use them as a gateway to *samadhi* (meditative absorption).

EXERCISE:

Close your eyes and listen very carefully to the sounds around you or concentrate on the sensations of your body. Notice this exercise affects your mind.

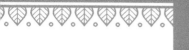

You Are the Light

1.36 OR INNER STABILITY IS
GAINED BY VISUALIZING A BRIGHT,
SORROWLESS LIGHT.

In Sutra 1.3 (see page 6), I mentioned that the spirit is like a steady light. It is beyond all fear, anxiety, and worry. Another method of calming the mind is to try to focus on this light either in the center of the forehead or in the center of the chest. You may not see or feel it at first, but with practice, this light will grow bigger and fill your entire being with illumination.

The sun is also a light that is always there whether you see it or not. In the same way that the light of the sun gives life to everything on Earth, the light of perception within you illuminates your world and brings it inside of you.

There is a practice called *trataka* where you focus on a dot on the wall, a candle, or any light source, like the moon, for some time without blinking. After you close your eyes, you can still see traces of the light inside of your mind's eye. If you continue to focus on this light, you will experience deep inner calm that you can reestablish anytime.

EXERCISE:
Try *trataka* with the flame of a candle or a dim lamp that is at eye level and two feet away from your face. Do not blink until your eyes tear up. Then close your eyes and focus on the light within.

Value of the Spiritual Master

1.37 OR THE MIND CAN BECOME STEADY BY CONTEMPLATING A MIND THAT IS FREE FROM ATTACHMENTS.

The mind takes on the qualities of whatever it focuses on. If you constantly watch scary movies, you are more likely to be scared in life or have scary dreams. If you experience natural and calm stimuli, your mind is more likely to feel natural and calm.

In many religious and spiritual communities, there is constant discussion of the actions and sayings of the masters of the tradition. The masters are like mentors who have spiritual achievements that are worth aspiring toward and cultivating. By the constant remembrance of them, the seeker's mind starts to take on the qualities of these noble people.

In the yoga tradition, the guru or spiritual master must be free from attachments and from negative qualities, like greed, hate, or envy. When I lived in yoga ashrams and practiced the yoga that was taught there, in almost every room there was a picture of the spiritual master to remind us of the steady wisdom, peace, and compassion that they had attained.

You can also choose to focus on a deity or a natural formation—like the sun, moon, or stars—if that gives you upliftment and tranquility.

EXERCISE:

Look at a picture of a guru or spiritual master for some time. Do you notice your mind becoming more steady?

Life Is Like a Dream

1.38 OR THE MIND CAN BECOME STEADY BY USING AS SUPPORT THE KNOWLEDGE ATTAINED FROM DREAMS AND DEEP SLEEP.

Focusing on your positive dreams from the previous night or on the stillness of deep sleep will calm your mind.

When you are sleeping, the conscious mind lets go of control, and many images are created from memories and experiences in the form of dreams. If you remember your dreams and analyze the images and symbols, you can start to understand the nature of your mind and the unfulfilled desires and background stressors of your life.

During the hours of deep (dreamless) sleep, you experience the same reality as the stillness of the spirit. By constantly identifying yourself as that witnessing spirit during the waking hours, you can maintain awareness even during these transitions in consciousness (between waking, dreaming, and deep sleep). Think of your spirit before going to sleep, and you may be able to "wake up" in the middle of a dream and do anything you like in that imaginary mental space.

EXERCISE:

For some time today, tell yourself that life is like a dream. How would you live your life if this were true? What things would you do differently? What things would you do the same way?

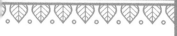

The Secret of Success

1.39 OR THE MIND BECOMES STILL
AND CONCENTRATED BY MEDITATING ON
ANYTHING YOU CHOOSE.

If none of the methods described thus far appeal to you, focus on any uplifting object or idea in order to calm the mind. It is important to choose something that is pleasing to you, like a flower or a loved one. What you shouldn't do is change the object every day.

You can start with a physical object or subtle idea, like the qualities of a great person. As your concentration develops further, you might focus on an energy center in the body or a more abstract idea, like love, truth, being, or infinity. The goal is to develop mental concentration. Then you can use the mind to penetrate deeply into any problem. When you choose not to think, you will experience inner stillness and joy.

By doing focused work or even as you read this book, the mind develops "one-pointedness." Successful people will tell you that their achievements are due to repeatedly bringing their focus back to a single subject. Multitasking in yoga and life will not lead you to mastery.

EXERCISE:

Think of an object or a quality that is spiritually uplifting for you. Close your eyes and sit quietly with this awareness for some time. If your mind wanders, mentally bring back the image or idea and start over again.

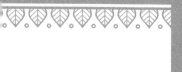

You Are Unlimited

1.40 THE YOGI'S MASTERY EXTENDS
FROM THE SMALLEST ATOM TO INFINITY.

When you have learned to calm and focus the mind, there is nothing that can stop you from achieving your goals. Any task is manageable if you view it as a succession of concrete moments.

When perception is refined and made sharp, it cannot be fooled by the imperfect senses. Yogis do not make unconscious choices due to conditioning or habits. They have complete control over their emotions. If you understand that other people are just trying to do their best, and that we are part of a global family, no one can disturb your peace. You can always respond with love and compassion.

When yogis meditate, it looks like they are not doing anything. Actually, they are penetrating into the deepest aspects of life and reality. Inside of them is the support of the higher self. They are prepared to efficiently deal with any challenge. By actively transforming experience into wisdom and insight, they are made confident and fearless. More importantly, they are able to attract and master anything they desire.

EXERCISE:

Make a list of all of the things you want to achieve or know in this lifetime. Think of the steps it will take you to get there and get started!

Sensitivity, Truth, and Power

1.41 THE MIND OF WEAKENED MODIFICATIONS, LIKE A FLAWLESS CRYSTAL, REFLECTS THE OBJECT ON WHICH IT RESTS, WHETHER THE OBJECT IS THE KNOWER, THE SENSES, OR THE OBJECT OF KNOWLEDGE. THIS BALANCED STATE IS CALLED *SAMADHI* (ENGROSSMENT OR ABSORPTION).

Do not confuse yoga with physical exercise or a pastime hobby that can be started and stopped whenever you choose. Yoga is primarily a psychology, which means that it is a wholehearted and consistent study of the self: mind, body, relationships, and environment.

As the sequence of lessons learned and realizations about life magnify, your concept of self evolves. Life choices become more significant as responsibility and sensitivity to the external world deepen. By refining your internal states, you will no longer feel powerless and pushed around by outside forces.

This book describes how to purify the mind and thereby cultivate and realize inner peace. The optimal mind is clear. It behaves like a spotless mirror that perfectly reflects to your soul the truth of anything put in front of it. With that foundation, your ability to know and understand anything (visible or invisible) is guaranteed.

REFLECTION:
How has your understanding of yoga practice changed since starting to read this book? Take a look back at the sutras in Book One and reflect on the ones that deepen your connection to your inner self.

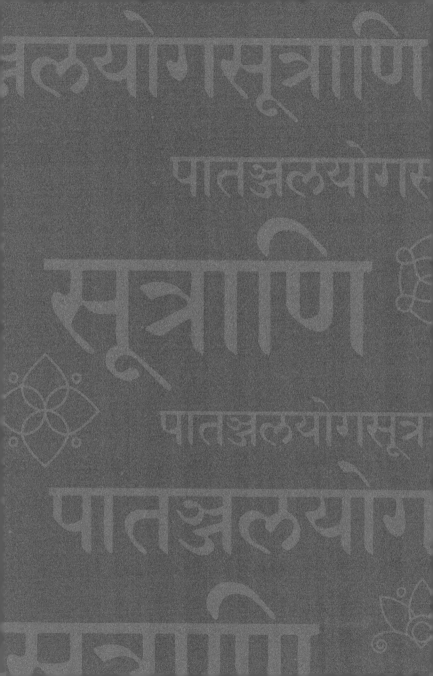

BOOK TWO

Purifying the Mind

The second book is known as the Book of Practice. Here, the root causes of suffering and the methods for removing them are explained. Spiritual growth is achieved by withdrawing our attachment to the material world.

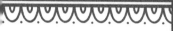

The Fire of Wisdom

2.1 DISCIPLINE (*TAPAS*), STUDY (*SVADYAYA*), AND SELF-SURRENDER (*ISHVARA PRANIDHANA*) ARE THE PURIFYING ACTIONS IN YOGA (KRIYA YOGA).

Book Two of *The Yoga Sutras* is dedicated to explaining the practices of yoga that purify the mind, body, senses, and ego. The three elements for transforming the will, intellect, and emotions are discipline, study, and self-surrender.

Tapas is developed by making any strong resolution and sticking to it. For example, when you sit still for a long period of time, a friction is created between the stillness and the habitual movements of the mind and body. This creates a psychic heat, which is also called *tapas*. It burns impurities in the body, rewires the brain, and builds spiritual power.

In order to know any process, *svadyaya* (study) is essential. You should study traditional texts and learn yoga mantras to be inspired and to redirect your thoughts. There are great yogis, however, who never read a book! Study of your own life and mind is also *svadyaya*.

Ishvara pranidhana is a realization that you are part of the wider universe and that you cannot control everything. It is also translated as "surrender to God." Yogis remain humble and know that they are connected to others and cannot accomplish everything by themselves.

EXERCISE:

The next time you experience physical or psychological pain, surrender to the experience, learn from it, and allow it to make you stronger.

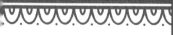

Yogic Skills and Perspective

2.2 THESE THREE ACTIONS (DISCIPLINE, STUDY, AND SELF-SURRENDER) HELP REDUCE OBSTACLES AND BRING ABOUT ENGROSSMENT (*SAMADHI*).

It is the constantly changing mind that inhibits our ability to see reality as it is. Left on its own, the mind is lazy or overactive and has prejudices that limit its understanding of things. *Samadhi* is the highest stage of concentration, outlined in Sutra 1.41 (see page 60). It is the goal of yoga and requires some preparation.

These three actions (Kriya Yoga) help develop detachment and interest in *samadhi*. They make you physically, mentally, and spiritually strong so that you no longer complain about life or make unconscious choices that you later regret.

Accepting pain from your resolutions (*tapas*), keeping a journal (*svadyaya*), and having faith in the path of yoga (*ishvara pranidhana*) eliminates distractions and weakens or removes psychological disturbances. Slowly, you develop a purified and focused mind that can look deeply into any problem. The result is clarity, strength, and confidence.

STORY:

My yoga students are not always interested in meditation at first. It is after months of practice and training in the history and philosophy of yoga that they start to seek more. Their inner and outer lives are transformed through meditation. All yoga practices help in the progression toward *samadhi*.

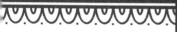

Chasing Happiness from the Outside

2.3 THE *KLESHAS* (MENTAL OBSTACLES) ARE IGNORANCE (*AVIDYA*), EGOISM (*ASMITA*), ATTACHMENT (*RAGA*), HATRED (*DVESHA*), AND THE FEAR OF DEATH (*ABHINIVESHA*).

You shouldn't confuse the five kleshas with the challenges listed in Sutra 1.30 (see page 38). These obstacles are more intellectual, emotional, and instinctive; they require a lot of effort and experience to overcome. The kleshas are the deep-seated psychological reasons for the constant instability of the untrained mind.

The spiritual path is not easy or accessible to people who are arrogant or have lots of desires. If you are filled with anger or fear of the unknown, then in meditation these fears might multiply or stop your progress. To have a firm belief and experience in the unchanging spirit within requires some reeducation and change of perspective. You must overcome the natural tendency for self-preservation and identification with the limited mind and body to excel in yoga.

REFLECTION:

Do you know anyone who is always making judgments about things or chasing stuff in the outside world? Do they seem happy with the clothes they have or the food they are eating, or are they never satisfied? Or do you know someone who is constantly looking at themselves in the mirror? How long do you think you could talk to them about spirituality?

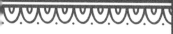

Spiritual Ignorance

2.4 IGNORANCE IS THE ROOT CAUSE OF THE OTHER OBSTACLES, WHICH CAN BE INACTIVE, WEAK, SOMETIMES ACTIVE, OR FULLY ACTIVE.

Many spiritual traditions teach that there is life after death and that your spirit is beyond the limitations of this life. The root of all suffering is to think that you are just this current mind and body and that everything is over when you die.

From the ignorance of not knowing your spiritual nature, you identify your true self with the body (egoism). From that thinking comes attraction (attachment) to pleasurable things. You cultivate an unhealthy repulsion (hatred) when other people or things get in the way of your pleasure. The ultimate manifestation of attachment and hatred is the clinging to life (or the fear of death).

These false ideas and reactions can be inactive, like in a child, or weak, like in an advanced yoga practitioner. They can be sometimes active, like in a beginning yoga practitioner, or fully active, like in the average person who makes no effort to control them. It takes constant practice to make the *kleshas* weaker or completely burned off.

REFLECTION:

What are some habits you have that might have been passed down from your family or you think are due to a past life? Are they completely gone or just waiting for the right opportunity to come back?

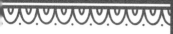

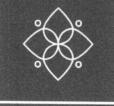

I Am Neither the Body nor the Mind

2.5 IGNORANCE (*AVIDYA*) IS MISTAKING THE TEMPORARY FOR THE PERMANENT, THE IMPURE AS PURE, PAIN FOR PLEASURE, AND NONSELF AS THE SELF.

Every moment that you bring your awareness to the present, don't you feel like what happened before is just not as important as right now? If you remember your higher self when your body or mind is in pain, doesn't the pain disappear for a moment? To lose connection to that pure inner self is ignorance.

The original (or root) ignorance is considering the self (the spirit), which is joyful, pure, and eternal, to be the nonself (the body/mind), which is painful, limiting, and temporary. The body is impure compared to the perfect spirit.

Spiritual ignorance is a state of mind, not a lack of knowledge. However, thinking that you know everything or making wrong judgments due to limited knowledge is also ignorance. Examples include jumping to conclusions, wishful thinking, or believing that disease is caused by anything other than your actions from either this life or past lives.

REFLECTION:

What are some things that you thought were pleasurable at first but actually were painful in the end?

Every Moment You Refresh

2.6 EGOISM (*ASMITA*) IS TO CONSIDER THE SELF AS THE MIND (AND BODY).

Our goal when studying the sutras is to develop spiritual perception—that is, a dual awareness of the changing body and mind along with the unchanging reality that is the spirit within. It is said that when enlightenment hits you, you laugh at the whole game of life. At that very moment, you realize that everything you obsessed about was not worth it and that the spirit was always with you and was not affected at all by material things.

In the unenlightened state, when you are hungry, you say to yourself, "I am hungry," but it is not you that is hungry; it is your body that is hungry. When you are angry, you think to yourself, "I am angry," but in reality it is just your mind that is angry for that moment. What actually remains after you eat or after the anger goes away?

Even during moments of hunger and anger, there is an unchanging spirit within you that is independently witnessing these passing states. You have momentarily misidentified the seer within you with the instruments of seeing, which are the mind, body, senses, and intelligence.

EXERCISE:
The next time you experience a moment of pain or difficulty, remind yourself that you are not the body or thoughts. Notice if that idea gives you strength, and meditate on that feeling. This feeling is you connected with the higher spiritual self.

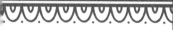

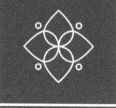

The Highest Bliss Is Within

2.7 ATTACHMENT (*RAGA*) COMES FROM
THE EXPERIENCE OF PLEASURE.

What you experience is a product of your actions and memories. How you react to experience results in more actions and memories. To perceive the world, you do not need to have a separate "I am" ego sense. As soon as you think, "I am seeing" or "I am experiencing," the ego pops up.

Then, experience is made into an object for the ego that brings pleasure or pain. When you experience something pleasant, it gets stored in your memory and you desire to experience it again—the result is attachment. You don't get attached to unpleasurable things.

This chain of events starts with the spirit getting linked to the senses or thoughts. Then you constantly think about pleasurable things and cannot detach your true self from the seeking of pleasure from outside. This process leads to the frustration of not getting what you want and feeling unfulfilled.

By reconnecting to the spirit within through yoga and meditation, you experience a bliss that is beyond any experience in nature or thought. It is a happiness that never ends and that reorganizes your expectations and desires. As you learn more about the sutras, accessing this bliss and happiness will become easier.

EXERCISE:

Make a list of all of the things that bring you happiness. Do they bring you lasting happiness? Can you be happy without them?

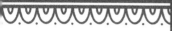

Do Not Overavoid

2.8 HATRED (*DVESHA*) COMES FROM THE EXPERIENCE OF PAIN.

The opposite of attachment (from attraction) is hatred (from repulsion). We are always running after things that bring us momentary happiness and running away from things that bring us pain. This constant push and pull is the reason outside things can never be ultimately satisfying.

However, pain is not always bad. When you make a resolution to cultivate tapas (discipline), there is an uncomfortableness that must be passed before purification can happen. It's like when you take medicine that doesn't taste good but ultimately cures you.

There is a healthy hatred that protects you from danger. For example, by instinct you might be afraid of snakes or aggressive dogs because you know that they can bite and even kill. What if you have a friend with a pet snake or dog? They love and enjoy them. Should you be afraid when you visit your friend?

It is not good to generalize and project anger and frustration on others without knowing the real situation. One bad experience should not shut you off from the rest of the world. Knowing the difference between healthy and unhealthy avoidance is the truth of this sutra.

EXERCISE:
The next time that you run into something you "hate" (like a kind of music or type of food), give it another try. Consider the culture behind it and allow your perspective to expand.

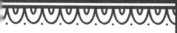

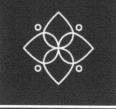

The Yogi Accepts Death

2.9 THE FEAR OF DEATH (*ABHINIVESHA*) IS A NATURAL TENDENCY, STRONG EVEN IN WISE PEOPLE.

In India, you can visit places where bodies are burned less than 24 hours after death. The experience of watching a body burn reminds you of how short life is and how nothing is left after the elements return to nature. The same thing happens when people are buried underground.

In all conscious living beings, the most basic instinct is the attachment to life and the fear of death. The more there is identification with the body and attachments and hatred, the more there is the insecurity of death. We think that all of the pleasures and pains of life are better than the void or unknown that comes after dying.

Even very old and sick people want to continue to live as long as they can. At the moment of death, a surge of unconscious reactions occurs that cannot be easily controlled. The truth is, death is a fantastic happening! It is a moment of great spiritual transformation and realization when the soul finally releases its attachment to the physical body.

EXERCISE:

Lie on the floor and imagine that you just died. Visualize your family and friends in mourning. It is a sad event, but remember that it's not that big of a deal because death is a part of life.

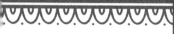

The Path to True Love

2.10 THE OBSTACLES ARE SUBTLE AND DISAPPEAR WHEN THE MIND RETURNS TO ITS ORIGINAL STATE.

Every moment, you have a choice to reconnect to your spirit. By doing so, your mind regains its original nature, which is calm and clear. Attachment and hatred are only momentary states of the mind, as is the "I am" ego thought.

The mind can stay pure by the practices of Kriya Yoga (discipline, study, and self-surrender) or by cultivating the opposites of the obstacles: nonattachment, nonhatred, understanding that "I am not the body/mind," and accepting the reality of death.

No person or thing in the world is trying to make you unhappy. You become unhappy due to expectations, laziness, overactivity, or reactions to the outside world. True happiness and joy come from knowing how to manage your mind and by realizing your true nature.

The source of life is love. Life is a creative expression and you are part of that infinite creativity. All obstacles are also part of the creative process of evolution and self-realization.

REFLECTION:

Do you think that in your core you are fear, hate, attachment, ego, ignorance, or love?

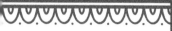

Practice Letting Go

2.11 THE STATES OF MIND PRODUCED BY OBSTACLES CAN BE AVOIDED BY MEDITATION.

There are various methods of meditation. As described in Book One, you can focus, for example, on the breath, a light, or a positive image. All of these methods help uproot and replace disturbing, painful, or negative thoughts. Likewise, it is helpful to meditate on phrases like "I am not the body" or "I am the eternal spirit."

Another kind of meditation is to simply observe what arises in the mind without reacting to it. When you close your eyes and a negative or positive thought comes in, just watch it. After some time, the thought will go away. Then maybe another thought will come. Just observe these thoughts and do not react.

With practice, you will notice (even when you are not meditating) the moment that fear, hatred, attachment, and ego arise within you. Become constantly watchful of these movements of the mind. By habit, the seeds of false identities and useless states of mind are burned away. Progress in the path of meditation leads to a pleasant inner experience and weakening of the mental obstacles.

EXERCISE:

One more method is to write down your thoughts before and during breaks in meditation. Let your mind unload its baggage for 10 minutes and see if inner stillness and solutions come to you.

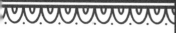

You Are What You Think and Do

2.12 THE STORE OF KARMAS (ACTIONS AND REACTIONS), WHICH BRING ABOUT EXPERIENCES IN PRESENT AND FUTURE LIVES, IS ROOTED IN THESE OBSTACLES (*KLESHAS*).

Your thoughts, likes, dislikes, and how you carry yourself in the company of others affect the choices you make and therefore the reality you experience—that is your karma. All actions and thoughts create subconscious impressions called *samskaras*. The strength of the five *kleshas* within you determines the strength of those impressions.

During meditation and dreams, these impressions come to the surface. In meditation, you actually witness and release these impressions from the deeper mind. The type of life that you experience upon rebirth is related to the unresolved *samskaras* and *kleshas* at the time of death.

The habits and tendencies that you have in this life are the result of your previous lives. For example, if you are interested in yoga more than others, it proves that in your past life you also practiced some yoga.

REFLECTION:

What experiences and natural skills in this life do you think have resulted from your past actions or a past life?

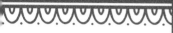

Life Is a University for the Soul

2.16 SUFFERING THAT HAS NOT YET
COME SHOULD BE AVOIDED.

All suffering is experienced for your own learning, and every soul is undergoing certain lessons as a result of karma. If you are (or were) a violent person, you experience more violence. These examples show that karma (and suffering) is both physical and psychological.

Skillful action is carried out with true knowledge and without selfish desire; it does not create painful karma but can lead to happiness instead. If you do volunteer work, for example, you are engaging in action to which you are not attached, and you feel great afterward.

From experience or from teachers, you can know which actions create bad results. If you have limitations and addictions, however, don't overreact. Take your time purging your karma and gaining wisdom from mistakes. It's good to remain detached from the body and mind because they are ultimately not the real you. However, always accept with humility the consequences of your actions. Be a spiritual warrior!

REFLECTION:

Think of some lessons you have learned from painful experiences. Have they changed the way you respond to situations and opportunities? Have you learned from them what to not repeat?

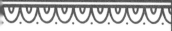

Motivation for Practice

2.17 THE CAUSE OF THAT AVOIDABLE PAIN IS THE JOINING OR ASSOCIATION OF THE SEER (SOUL) WITH THE SEEN (MIND, BODY, AND NATURE).

The ups and downs of life recreate cravings and desires that keep us unsatisfied. Isn't it frustrating trying to find permanent happiness in the objects of the world, which are by nature temporary? Those things we work hard to get we are afraid to lose. Also, as long as there is a body, there is going to be old age and disease. It seems like almost everything eventually causes pain.

These realizations are necessary to start the yogic path with enthusiasm. Without suffering and the belief that there may be a way out, what else would motivate someone to follow the path of yoga in earnest? This book is the outline of that path.

The good news is that the soul is always pure and free; it does not suffer. It appears to feel pleasure and pain because of its momentary association with the mind, body, and senses. With the right attitude and perspective toward the outside world, you can become like the lotus flower in muddy water—established in the purity of the spirit and unaffected by outside circumstances.

REFLECTION:
Have you ever felt better by not doing something than by doing it?

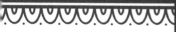

The Purpose of Nature

2.18 NATURE HAS THE QUALITIES OF CLARITY (*SATTVA*), ACTIVITY (*RAJAS*), AND HEAVINESS (*TAMAS*). IT ALSO INCLUDES THE ELEMENTS AND THE SENSES. ITS PURPOSE IS TO PROVIDE EXPERIENCE AND LIBERATION FOR THE SOUL.

Everything in nature, like the mind, body, and objects, is made up of three *gunas* (*sattva*, *rajas*, and *tamas*). When the mind is *sattvic*, it is in its original nature and has a steady rhythm. It is well balanced and able to see things clearly.

Rajas is the quality of movement in an object. When you eat spicy foods, the mind gets agitated, which is its *rajasic* state. *Tamas* is the solidity of an object, or when something is not moving. When you fall asleep at night, the mind transitions into a *tamasic* mode, where it feels heavy and stops moving.

The elements are earth, water, fire, air, and space. The senses are smell, taste, vision, touch, and hearing. Karma links the *gunas* of the mind with the elements of the body and senses. Through life, nature pulls you in for experience and learning, only to eventually push you away toward the path to ultimate freedom and liberation of the soul.

REFLECTION:

Are you noticing your evolution and increased control as you learn and experience more of life?

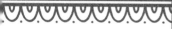

What the Sutras Have Given Us So Far

2.28 FROM THE PRACTICES OF YOGA, IMPURITIES ARE DESTROYED AND SPIRITUAL WISDOM ARISES, LEADING TO ENLIGHTENED VISION (DISCRIMINATIVE DISCERNMENT).

The impurities are the negative *samskaras* (subconscious impressions) and the *kleshas* (ignorance, ego, attachment, hatred, and the fear of death). We can also include the distractions from Sutra 1.30 (see page 38): disease, dullness, doubt, carelessness, laziness, craving, false perception, failure to reach firm ground, and slipping from the ground gained.

The practices of yoga that we have discussed so far include Kriya Yoga (discipline, study, and self-surrender), constant remembrance of the distinction between the soul and nature (which includes the mind, body, and senses), and the techniques to keep the mind calm in Sutras 1.32 through 1.39 (see pages 42–56).

From understanding and practicing these elements of yoga, the mind becomes calm and your intuitive intelligence increases in the form of spiritual wisdom. The enlightened vision that we seek is to realize that the soul is always free and full of joy, and it should not be confused with karma or the passing states of the mind and body.

REFLECTION:

Do you understand everything so far and have faith in yourself? At this point, feel free to revisit past sutras in order to deepen your understanding of the concepts.

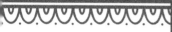

Ashtanga Yoga

2.29 THE EIGHT LIMBS (OR STEPS) OF YOGA ARE *YAMA* (THINGS NOT TO DO), *NIYAMA* (THINGS TO DO), *ASANA* (STEADY POSTURE), *PRANAYAMA* (BREATH CONTROL), *PRATYAHARA* (WITHDRAWING THE SENSES INWARD), *DHARANA* (CONCENTRATION), *DHYANA* (MEDITATION), AND *SAMADHI* (ABSORPTION).

Now Patanjali lists very specific things to do and not do, followed by a very systematic way of steadying the body, its energies, the senses, and the mind. These eight steps are called Ashtanga Yoga, or the eight-limbed path. It is a very practical system that makes deep meditation possible and therefore helps remove the obstacles and impurities.

The goal is to become established in that absorbed state of *samadhi* mentioned in Sutra 1.41 (see page 60). Learning how to focus the mind on any subject with concentration, meditation, and absorption will also allow it to achieve great abilities and insights that are described in the sutras of Book Three.

Although they are described as steps that you need to do one at a time, it is possible to experience them out of order. For example, when we watch a movie, we feel like we become one with the characters—a lower form of *samadhi*.

REFLECTION:

How would your life be improved if you could control all of your habits and focus your mind for long periods of time?

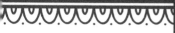

Living Peacefully in Society

2.30 *YAMA* CONSISTS OF *AHIMSA* (NONVIOLENCE), *SATYA* (NOT LYING/TRUTHFULNESS), *ASTEYA* (NOT STEALING), *BRAHMACHARYA* (NOT HAVING SEX/CELIBACY), AND *APARIGRAHA* (NONPOSSESSIVENESS).

Imagine you hurt others, lied all the time, stole from people, had multiple sexual partners, and hoarded lots of things. What would happen when you tried to meditate? You would have violent and desire-filled thoughts in your mind. You would worry if people found out about your stealing and lies. This way of living is the opposite of the yogic ideal.

For steady progress on the spiritual path, it's best to develop equal love for everyone and not be greedy. When you exaggerate or pretend to be something you are not, your inner conscience will remain disturbed. These ideals help you keep smooth and simple relationships with others so that in meditation you feel unattached and lighthearted.

The most important of the *yamas* is nonviolence. From slowly mastering the *yamas*, you will no longer experience conflict around you, everything you say will happen, anything you need will come to you, you will be physically powerful, and you will know the reason for your birth.

EXERCISE:

For one month, try not to buy anything that you don't absolutely need. At the end of the month, examine if you even remember any of the things you wanted to buy.

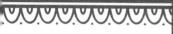

Timeless Teachings

2.31 THESE GREAT VOWS ARE UNIVERSAL AND APPLY TO ANY SOCIAL CLASS, PLACE, TIME, OR SITUATION.

Some people think that it is okay to break a couple of the *yamas* sometimes. Maybe you will go to a nonvegetarian home and feel that you should eat food that came from the killing of animals. Or you feel that it's okay to kill an insect that comes into your house.

People may lie when engaged with or participating in politics or are violent when they play some sports. Some people make their living by gambling or through tricky financial techniques. Others may not be able to follow a life of strict celibacy due to emotional needs. These situations make it harder to truly attain the fantastic and profound results described later.

Each person has their own unique karmas; we have the freedom to live the life we choose. By Patanjali's standards, in order to go all the way on the path, these rules are essential and universal to those who have succeeded. The high ideals described in this book are for full-time yogis who seek infinite bliss and independence from the physical world. In any lifetime, we can practice yoga to the best of our ability and pick it up again in the next life.

REFLECTION:

Which of the *yamas* seems the easiest for you to maintain? Which of them seems the hardest to maintain?

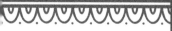

How to Be Strong and Happy

2.32 *NIYAMA* CONSISTS OF *SAUCHA* (INTERNAL AND EXTERNAL PURITY), *SANTOSHA* (CONTENTMENT), *TAPAS* (DISCIPLINE), *SVADYAYA* (STUDY), AND *ISHVARA PRANIDHANA* (SELF-SURRENDER).

The *yamas* and *niyamas* are like an extension of the Kriya Yoga explained in Sutra 2.1 (see page 64). *Niyama* includes the three elements of *tapas*, *svadyaya*, and *ishvara pranidhana* and adds purity and contentment. These elements do not require other people in order to be practiced.

To be pure refers to cleanliness but also to making an effort to purify the body and mind. Yogis employ various practices to this end, like eating only natural foods and occasionally fasting in order to rid the body of toxins. Contentment means being happy with less. Cleanliness and contentment free energy for meditation.

By these practices, you can master your body and senses and become more inclined toward celibacy. They weaken or destroy the impurities and make you more joyful and cheerful always. Through these disciplines, you can achieve any mental ideal you choose and safely progress toward *samadhi*.

EXERCISE:
Try not showering for a day, wearing dirty clothes, or fasting for a short time. Notice how your energy changes.

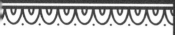

We Are a Global Family

2.33 WHEN DISTURBING NEGATIVE THOUGHTS (AGAINST THE *YAMAS* AND *NIYAMAS*) COME, THINK OF THEIR OPPOSITE (*PRATIPAKSHA BHAVANA*).

Developing the positive qualities of the *yamas* and *niyamas* removes mental and emotional disturbances. If you have a thought that is against them, find the selfish desire or *samskaras* (subconscious impressions) that might be the cause. Maybe it is just the changing *gunas* (three states of nature) that are causing your mood to fluctuate.

To spread positive energy to everyone around you and to cultivate discipline are beyond any short-lived experience of pleasure, fame, or wealth. When you have unpleasant thoughts or weakening of self-discipline, you are only hurting yourself.

If someone cuts you off in traffic, think to yourself about a time you might have made the same mistake, and send them compassion instead of anger. If anyone hurts you, have patience and send them love. Always try to think of others in a nonviolent way, like a family member or another soul who is just trying to do their best.

EXERCISE:

Are you judgmental or angry? Try becoming kinder and more accepting. It will change how others see and interact with you.

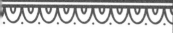

Easeful, Peaceful, and Useful

2.46 ASANA IS A STEADY AND COMFORTABLE POSTURE.

Most people cannot sit still for long periods of time. Either their mind won't allow it or their body gives them pain. For this reason, there are a variety of yoga poses that calm the nerves and develop an easeful body by positively affecting digestion, hormonal health, and musculoskeletal tone.

Asana literally means "sitting," so it can be done even on a chair. During meditation, it is important to keep the spine straight and upright for long periods. If you practice yoga poses before meditating, your breathing will be deeper and you will feel more calm.

A lean or perfectly healthy body is not a measure of success in yoga. The greatest yogis were not gymnasts but were masters of concentration, compassion, and wisdom through connection to the spirit. The goal is beyond building a strong and beautiful body, which could increase the ego (identification of your true spiritual nature with the temporary mind and body).

Remember that *asana* is only one of the eight limbs of yoga.

REFLECTION:

Do you know anyone with great spiritual energy but not a "perfect body"? Notice how you can see and feel their energy regardless of their appearance. Use this knowledge to inspire you on your own journey.

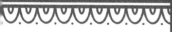

Become Like Space

2.47 *ASANA* IS PERFECTED BY RELAXATION OF EFFORT AND MEDITATING ON INFINITY.

During *asana* practice, you may experience some discomfort at first. Not all poses are suitable for everybody, so it is important to have a good teacher who does not encourage competitiveness or straining. You should feel comfortable and experience inner joy during and after yoga practice. If you push too hard, the body will record the pain and rebel against you.

The mind takes the shape of whatever it focuses on. If you focus on infinite space, then your mind and body will take the form of infinite spaciousness. They will become so quiet that you will forget you even have a body or mind! As the mind and breath become more tranquil in the poses, you will notice that the bodily functions harmonize and the body itself becomes less stiff.

If your yoga practice always requires strenuous physical effort, when will your striving end? When will you go into the mind and address the sources of suffering? Real yoga creates space and expands your concept of self. Yoga reunites you with your innate happiness, which is your birthright.

EXERCISE:

Try one simple yoga pose and imagine that you are infinite, invisible, and made of vast space. Meditate on this infinitude.

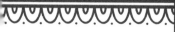
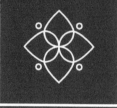

In All Conditions, You Remain Unchanged

2.48 FROM THE MASTERY OF *ASANA*, ONE WILL NOT BE DISTURBED BY PAIRS OF OPPOSITES (LIKE HOT AND COLD).

Asana is a method to establish equilibrium in the body, mind, and senses. Through stillness, energy is conserved and the mind is not distracted during meditation.

To master *asana* means to be able to stay in one pose without effort, trembling, or strain for over two hours. This ability requires a lot of consistent practice and willpower. *Asana*, therefore, is also a psychological and emotional posture. Your attitude toward life should be steady and comfortable.

When the body learns stillness, the mind also gains stability. Through *asana* practice, your mood becomes steady. You will not overreact to sadness or happiness, to blame or praise, or to wealth or poverty. These various experiences are passing and should not overshadow the brilliance of your spirit.

My friends are always surprised by my ability to swim in cold ocean water. It's really a question of mind over matter or harnessing spiritual heat (*tapas*).

EXERCISE:

The next time you experience a slightly uncomfortable room temperature, focus on its impermanence and see if you can find calm and acceptance.

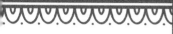

Cultivating Life Force Energy

2.49 *PRANAYAMA* IS THE REGULATION OF THE MOVEMENTS OF INHALATION AND EXHALATION. IT SHOULD BE PRACTICED WHEN *ASANA* IS ACCOMPLISHED.

It is the *prana* (life force) that allows movement, sensing, thinking, and knowing. We get *prana* from food, water, air, and the sun. The *prana* that enters the body travels through subtle channels that regulate the movement of energy within.

When you have made the body still by *asana*, the next spontaneous movement that you notice is the breath; it is intimately connected to your emotions and energy levels. For this reason, yogis have very elaborate practices for regulating and stabilizing the breath. Working with the breath is described in Sutra 1.34 (see page 46). There are even practices for clearing the nasal passages with saltwater or by using a thread.

Prana is wasted by inefficient actions like overthinking, overworking, overeating, or overtalking. It is cultivated by *pranayama*, spending time in nature, practicing *asanas* (poses) slowly, and consuming fresh water and food.

EXERCISE:

Ask your yoga teacher to teach you alternate nostril breathing. Try it for five minutes before meditation and before going to sleep for better rest and dreams.

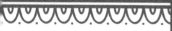

Mastering the Breath

2.50 *PRANAYAMA* IS EXTERNAL, INTERNAL, OR SUPPRESSED. WHEN REGULATED BY PLACE, TIME, AND NUMBER, THE BREATH BECOMES LONG AND SUBTLE.

Prana means breath or life force, and *ayama* means lengthening, expansion, regulation, restraint, or control. In the advanced stages of practice, the yogi learns how to hold the breath. By doing so, the mind is made completely still.

Breath retention can happen after the exhale or after the inhale, or breathing can spontaneously stop on its own. There are a few internal energy locks, called *bandhas*, that help achieve this effect. Dietary and lifestyle observances are involved, so proper instruction is necessary. Some yogis can remain breathless for a week or longer!

In this sutra, the "place" is either external (feeling air flow from the tip of the nose to the upper lip) or internal (visualizing energy moving throughout the body). "Time" refers to how long the breath is held or how long it takes to exhale and inhale air. The "number" is how many times *pranayama* is practiced.

EXERCISE:

Count how many seconds you inhale. Try to exhale for double that count. Visualize energy moving up the spine on the inhale and down on the exhale.

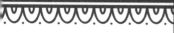

The Breath of Life

2.52 AS A RESULT OF *PRANAYAMA*, THE COVER OF THE INNER LIGHT OF KNOWLEDGE IS REMOVED.

When *pranayama* is practiced correctly, it heals the mind and the body—especially the nervous system. By *pranayama*, digestion is improved and breathing becomes more efficient. Consequently, a lightness is felt in the body and mind. It is the ultimate energy conservation. A yogi might take only one or two breaths per minute, whereas the average person breathes 14 times a minute.

There are stages to advanced breath control. Holding the breath is very dangerous because it can cause unconsciousness or irregularities in the heartbeat. To play with the breath in this way is to face the fear of death. Yogis who master these techniques experience consistently steady mental and physical energy and the unfolding of psychic faculties.

There is a form of *pranayama* called "the skull-shining breath," which creates the appearance of light in the center of the forehead when the eyes are closed. Coming in contact with subtle life force energies illuminates what drives our behavior and reactions to things.

REFLECTION:

Think about a dog and a turtle. Which one breathes faster? Which one moves faster? Which one lives longer?

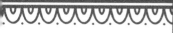

Gateway to the Inner Yoga

2.53 THROUGH *PRANAYAMA*, THE MIND BECOMES READY FOR CONCENTRATION.

Pranayama is the gateway to the higher practices of yoga. It increases the clarity (*sattva*) of the mind and burns up laziness (*tamas*) and overactivity (*rajas*). It is like a meditation practice in itself that stills the movements of the mind and makes it one-pointed.

When you diligently and patiently practice *pranayama*, your capacity for inner stillness and concentration increases. It gives you energy to keep your spine straight and mind alert. Controlling *prana* makes it easier to separate your ego ("I am" sense) from the body so you can focus on just the mind (or beyond).

How you manage your life energies determines your emotions and how well you can control your thoughts. It is not always necessary to practice *pranayama* before meditation, but it helps your ability to form steady and sharp mental images.

> **EXERCISE:**
>
> To improve your experience of meditation and integration, try some yoga poses first to remove fatigue and restlessness. Then do a few minutes of breath awareness or alternate nostril breathing. Finally, focus on one spot of light in the center of the forehead and hold the stillness within.

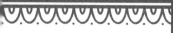

The Outer World Disappears

2.54 *PRATYAHARA* OCCURS WHEN THE
SENSES DISREGARD THE OBJECTS OF
THE OUTSIDE WORLD AND FOLLOW THE
DIRECTION OF THE MIND INWARD.

When you practice *pranayama* or meditation, at first you still hear the sounds in the room or feel your clothes against your body. You may also have various thoughts about the surroundings, like the temperature of the room or light on your eyelids. Eventually, you stop noticing these things. That moment is *pratyahara*.

The experience is similar to when you go to sleep at night. Right before you forget about the world and go into your inner self, there are a few moments when you are still aware of the outside world. Suddenly the person snoring next to you or the sound of the clock disappears.

What is happening is that the *prana*, which usually causes the senses to experience the outside world, is redirected inward for rest, healing, and introspection. Even during *asana*, the same inward process is happening. All the practices of yoga are interconnected and promote the inward movement of energy and awareness.

EXERCISE:
Set a timer for 10 minutes and try the yoga pose called *savasana*. Stay aware as your body and mind become relaxed; you will experience *pratyahara*.

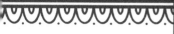

Harness the Power of the Senses

2.55 FROM THE PRACTICE OF *PRATYAHARA*, SUPREME MASTERY OVER THE SENSES IS GAINED.

Imagine if every time you saw a piece of cake, you had to eat it. Or imagine not being able to just wait and do nothing for a while. There is a restlessness in many people. Especially with cell phones, our society has become addicted to constant sensory stimulation. Always watching videos or listening to music makes us a slave to the senses. We are constantly searching outside for gratification and entertainment, which is a big problem of our current era.

Yogis will often eat plain food or fast for some time in order to gain control over their senses. By conserving energy and focusing within, they can harness healing energy and develop the power to concentrate on anything they choose (inside or outside).

With every experience of *pratyahara* (sensory withdrawal), the independence of the spirit from the mind and body is reestablished. The senses follow the *prana*. When the mind, body, and breath are under control, the senses are also under control. Through yoga, we become the master of our senses.

EXERCISE:

For one week, give up that one food or habit that constantly pulls your awareness outward. If you feel addicted to your cell phone, give yourself at least a few hours a day without it.

BOOK THREE

Stabilizing the Mind

In the third book, known as the
Book of Spiritual Powers, we will explore
the insights that are possible through
yogic concentration.

The Concentrated Mind

3.1 *DHARANA* (CONCENTRATION) IS HOLDING THE MIND ON A SINGLE OBJECT OR IDEA.

The first five limbs of yoga prepare us to focus our attention on just the mind. We are learning not to suppress our emotions and desires but to bring them under our conscious control. Through *asana* (steady posture), *pranayama* (breath control), and *pratyahara* (sensory withdrawal), we are able to redirect our awareness away from the outside world. What about working with the mind directly? That's where *dharana* comes in.

Dharana is the effort to concentrate the mind. It's natural for the mind to resist focusing at first. As you practice concentrating on one thing, like your breath or a flower, you will find your mind becoming more still and relaxed. It will resist less and less as it grows calmer. You may find that your breath and body naturally relax too.

By repeating the effort to concentrate, the quiet gaps between thoughts will grow. After spending time in this quiet space, you may notice answers and creative solutions arising more easily in your daily life.

EXERCISE:

Set a timer for five minutes. Close your eyes and choose an object or idea to focus on. Allow your mind to relax and gently bring it back whenever it wanders. How do you feel after this exercise?

The Engaged and Peaceful Mind

3.2 WHEN *DHARANA* (CONCENTRATION) IS UNINTERRUPTED, THAT STATE IS *DHYANA* (MEDITATION).

For a mind new to concentration, sometimes one idea will lead you to another until you end up nowhere near where you started. At other times, an image from the past or a thought about what you have to do later might come up. Between these breaks in concentration, you keep reminding yourself, "Oh yeah, I'm supposed to be concentrating."

Instead of battling with the mind, consider hearing it out. If a thought keeps interrupting your concentration, pause and consider it. Write it down so you can come back to it later.

Slowly, after processing these surface thought ripples, you will start to penetrate deeper into the subconscious mind. You'll uncover and let go of subtle attachments and the habits of the wandering mind.

Eventually, you will need to make less and less effort to concentrate. When your mind experiences fewer interruptions, you'll glide into a tranquil, peaceful state called *dhyana*.

REFLECTION:

The next time you are fully engaged with something, notice if it feels like time passes really fast. If it does, you are in a state of meditation.

Real Knowing

3.3 WHEN ONLY THE TRUTH OF THE OBJECT MEDITATED UPON IS EXPERIENCED, AS IF THERE IS NO SEPARATE MIND, THAT STATE IS *SAMADHI* (ABSORPTION).

As you progress in meditation, the secrets of yoga are revealed.

Imagine that you are alone in a field. You pick up a blade of grass and look at it very intensely. Slowly, you will forget about everyone and anything else in the world. Because your body is still, your breathing will slow down. As you focus, everything around this blade of grass will disappear. You have reached the stage of *pratyahara* (sensory withdrawal).

Keep concentrating on this blade of grass and you will begin to see its smallest details. After many more minutes, you will stop thinking about the details, and your mind will naturally be glued to the object. At this point you have reached the stage of *dhyana* (meditation).

Do you know what happens if you keep going for an hour or two? You become that blade of grass! You will know everything about that object.

REFLECTION:

How does a music student become a composer or a cooking student a chef?

Perfect Control

3.4 WHEN *DHARANA* (CONCENTRATION), *DHYANA* (MEDITATION), AND *SAMADHI* (ABSORPTION) ARE PRACTICED TOGETHER ON ONE OBJECT, IT IS CALLED *SAMYAMA* (PERFECT CONTROL OF MENTAL CONCENTRATION).

Every object that we use in our modern life first came from a thought in the mind of someone. They most likely spent a lot of time planning how this thing would be used by others and what problems it would solve. Think about a car, how many parts it has, and how many calculations must have gone into designing the final product. At each step of its creation, a lot of thinking was involved.

If you want to know an object or to find the solution to a problem, you must focus deeply. The type of focus that yogis develop is unique because they learn to make their body, breath, and senses completely still before going into the mind, which is more powerful than we commonly appreciate.

Samyama is just another name for the three practices of concentration, meditation, and absorption applied together. We attain a variety of insights and abilities by applying *samyama* to various activities and experiences. Those teachings are the subject of Book Three of *The Yoga Sutras*.

EXERCISE:

Focus on your body. How many processes are going on there right now? Keep focusing until the body starts to communicate with you. It will reveal more the longer you are able to focus.

From External to Internal

3.7 THESE THREE (*DHARANA, DHYANA, AND SAMADHI*) ARE MORE INTERNAL THAN THE PREVIOUS LIMBS (*YAMA, NIYAMA, ASANA, PRANAYAMA,* AND *PRATYAHARA*).

The different steps in the eight-limbed path are organized in order of subtlety and introversion. The first five purify the actions, body, *prana*, and senses. *Dharana*, *dhyana*, and *samadhi*, the final three, purify and strengthen the mind and intellect.

It is easy to recognize and make changes that affect the first five steps. The final three, which deal only with the mind and intellect, are more subtle and internal. Two advanced yogis may not appear very different from the outside, but what they have accomplished on the inner dimensions of spirit and wisdom can vary greatly.

From their actions and thoughts, we may be able to understand something, but many advanced yogis do not talk about their inner research, realizations, and capabilities. Others are unknown to the public because they are practicing in remote places.

REFLECTION:
How can you tell a real yogi from an insincere one? Is it possible to tell by observing someone?

Without Seed

3.8 EVEN *SAMYAMA* IS EXTERNAL COMPARED TO SEEDLESS (*NIRBIJA*) *SAMADHI*.

Sutras 1.17 (see page 34) and 1.18 (see page 36) describe two types of *samadhi*, called *samprajnata* and *asamprajnata*. In *samprajnata samadhi*, the yogi gains knowledge of an object spontaneously and intuitively when the mind becomes one with it.

After various *samprajnata* experiences, a*samprajnata samadhi* occurs when the object that is used for meditation comes from the subconscious mind or from past experiences or impressions (*samskaras*). Instead of picking an object and gaining knowledge about that thing, you allow what remains in the psyche to come up and use it to transcend the mind.

In both of these *samadhi*s, there is an object (or seed) used to get into the *samadhi* state. Going further on the path requires that knowledge gained is transcended and that even the roots of the ego (which the *samskaras* represent) are removed or wiped out.

Nirbija samadhi is the last stage of a*samprajnata*, when the mind completely dissolves and no more impressions remain. *Nirbija* in Sanskrit literally means "without seed." The sense of a separate ego is completely gone. It does not return. In that state you no longer identify with the mind or body.

EXERCISE:

Contemplate the seer within you, which is unchanging. Remember that the truth of your soul is always present. Connect with it now.

Letting Go

3.9 WHEN YOU RELEASE AN OUTGOING THOUGHT BY THE HABIT OF SUPPRESSION, YOU EXPERIENCE *NIRODHA PARINAMA* (MODIFICATION OF CONTROL).

By observing the *yamas* and *niyamas*, and becoming a witness to the mind, you will spontaneously release many thoughts and feelings. In this way, the yogi is at one with the freshness of each moment. You are able to refresh yourself easily and connect to the present moment as it is.

Each time that the mind becomes still, clear, and focused is a moment of *nirodha*. As you experience and practice *nirodha* during meditation or even in your day, you are creating a new habit of stillness and redirecting the attention inward.

Then, during meditation, it is easier to let go of thoughts. You notice a thought arise like a bubble that immediately bursts without any effort. The subconscious mind still has material in it, but you can observe and release it without reacting. The moment of control and stillness is called *nirodha parinama*.

At this point, the mind is moving from a preoccupation with thoughts to freedom from thoughts. Staying in this state for as long as possible is the purpose of meditation.

EXERCISE:
As you meditate, notice the exact moment when a thought arises, and let it pop like a bubble.

Calm

3.10 WITH THE RESTRAINT OF
IMPRESSIONS, A CALM FLOW ARISES.

The most pleasant state of the mind is when it is still and calm. Usually we have lots of different thoughts, emotions, attachments, and desires that keep us from fully experiencing the present moment and the wonder of being alive.

Through meditation, a sustained balance and harmony is reestablished within our being, and we can maintain a state of inner peace at all times. This state of being takes practice and nonattachment. As the mind becomes more focused and deeper levels of concentration develop, it becomes more efficient and our lives start to change.

By staying mindful and developing the habit of letting go of rising impressions, our perspective changes and life becomes like a video game. We don't allow fear or thoughts of the past or future linger in our mind. This practice eventually allows for effortless entry into the *samadhi* state, where we can acquire knowledge and realize the light of the soul.

Yogis move in the world gracefully and confidently. Their optimism and joy are untouched by the difficulties of life.

REFLECTION:

Notice when you feel the most calm. What did you do or not do in order to get there? How does that state affect your perception of life?

No Turning Back

3.11 WHEN THE SCATTERED STATE OF MIND SUBSIDES AND THE ONE-POINTED MIND ARISES, IT IS CALLED *SAMADHI PARINAMA* (MODIFICATION OF ABSORPTION).

The mind exists in one of five states: dull, restless, distracted, one-pointed, or restrained.

The distracted mind is occupied by multiple objects, like in the untrained state. Depending on past tendencies and how you respond to them, you may be very easily distracted and allow the first thing that comes to your mind to pull you away, or you might be able to bring your focus back for a moment.

If you are patient in meditation, there comes a moment when suddenly your mind will change its character and become absorbed in itself or an object. This experience is like jumping off of a cliff or riding a roller coaster when there is no turning back, and you are effortlessly absorbed and engaged.

At that moment, the mind has changed into the one-pointed state. This change happens during the transition between *dhyana* (meditation) and *samadhi* (absorption). *Samadhi* is like a trance during which there is no ego, only a peaceful flow of presence and truth.

EXERCISE:

Try staring at something for a couple of minutes. At first your mind will jump around. When it has finally settled on just that thing, tell yourself, "Aha—*samadhi parinama!*"

One-Pointedness

3.12 IN *SAMADHI*, WHEN THE RELEASED PAST IMPRESSION AND THE ARISING PRESENT IMPRESSION IN THE MIND ARE THE SAME, IT IS CALLED *EKAGRATA PARINAMA* (MODIFICATION OF ONE-POINTEDNESS).

Once you reach a state of effortless absorption and there is no longer a tendency to run after other objects, you notice that there is only one object in your awareness. Another way to describe this state is to say that every image you see in your mind is similar to the next. Time appears to stop; this moment is *ekagrata parinama.*

I remember one afternoon practicing yoga on the beach. After my *asana* practice, I momentarily looked at the sun on the horizon and then closed my eyes. I sat for *pranayama* and meditation. My breathing became deeper and slower. I stopped the breathing practices and suddenly I could not feel my body. Everything became silent. I forgot all about myself and my surroundings.

Maintaining my awareness on the center of the forehead, I could still see traces of the sun there. It was like an orange ball surrounded by darkness. I continued to focus for a few minutes and noticed that the orange ball got bigger. Then there was only light and bliss.

EXERCISE:

Try meditating in the way I did on the beach. Look at an object and then close your eyes and visualize it. If you have to, open your eyes to look again and return to focusing inward.

Transformations

3.13 BY THESE MODIFICATIONS (OF *NIRODHA*, *SAMADHI*, AND *EKAGRATA*), THE CHANGES IN THE CHARACTERISTIC, TIME STATE, AND CONDITION OF OBJECTS AND SENSE ORGANS ARE UNDERSTOOD.

Everything is constantly changing on three levels. For example, when the mind changes from one-pointedness (*ekagrata*) to the arrested state (*nirodha*), its characteristic changes. The "characteristic" is the general shape and functioning of a thing. Another example is melting a metal spoon and shaping the metal into a key. Objects and their functions can transform.

The second level is the "time state"—past, present, or future. For example, when the mind changes from the one-pointed state to the arrested state, the arrested state shifts from the nonexisting future to existing in the present.

The "condition" is the age or strength of an object. For example, the strength of a multipointed mind weakens as it becomes one-pointed.

As the mind experiences these changes, perception of objects of the world through the senses also changes. As yogis learn to master the mind, they are able to master the elements and the senses.

EXERCISE:

Focus on an object in the room that you are in. Think about its function and age. As your mind becomes more focused, can you experience its relative function and age change?

Your Essence Remains

3.14 THE BACKGROUND ESSENCE STAYS THE SAME IN ALL STATES (PAST, PRESENT, AND FUTURE).

Consciousness is awareness, or the ability to know or perceive. It is also another term for the spirit or your true self. Each of us has this consciousness within us. When consciousness interacts with nature, experience happens. At any moment, however, consciousness can also separate itself from perception of the outside world.

The *gunas* of nature (states of heaviness, activity, and clarity) constantly affect the mind, senses, and objects, but nature itself does not change—neither does consciousness. When you go to sleep at night, you are reminded of this separation between you and the outside world.

Even as the body gets old, or your hearing and vision get worse with age, your essence inside does not change. The same natural energies are out there that constantly transform the mind and *samskaras* (impressions), but these are all part of the outside chain of cause and effect. It's the witness that recreates worldly experience in every moment.

The yogic view is that intention and attitude have an effect on our perception and what we experience. That force is the power of spirit.

REFLECTION:

Think about how you have mentally and physically changed throughout your life. Now think about your essence or the witness within. Has it changed?

Little Changes Create Big Changes

3.15 THE DIFFERENCE IN THE ORDER OF EVENTS CREATES DIFFERENT TRANSFORMATIONS (IN MIND AND OBJECTS).

Everything that happens is due to small changes in very small moments of time. This idea explains why, if you want something to change in your life, you need to make a little effort every day. For example, to experience the effects of exercise or meditation, you have to work on it every day.

First you must know that there is a possibility for change and to study the steps involved. Are there other people who have succeeded? What do they say?

When I started practicing yoga *asana*s, I had very tight hip muscles. It was difficult for me to sit still without pain in my knees or lower back. Also, I used to be very judgmental and competitive; plus, I would always stay out late with my friends. As I continued to read about the yogic lifestyle, including diet and regular practice, changes started to happen in my body and mind.

There is nothing that is not in the flow of change and that cannot be changed. With the application of willpower and effort, you can transform the habits of the mind, body, and personality.

REFLECTION:
Have you noticed your thinking and behaviors change slowly over time?

Seeing the Past and Future

3.16 BY *SAMYAMA* ON THE THREE KINDS OF MENTAL TRANSFORMATIONS (*NIRODHA*, *SAMADHI*, AND *EKAGRATA*), KNOWLEDGE OF THE PAST AND THE FUTURE ARISES.

Now Patanjali starts to describe the supernatural powers that yogis can attain from deep concentration on objects and ideas. If you practice concentration, meditation, and absorption on the three mental transformations, you can penetrate into the nature of time and cause and effect.

During the change to the one-pointed state (*ekagrata parinama*), the object of perception stays the same for some time. In *samadhi parinama*, a particular set of properties is focused on, and there is no change. When *nirodha parinama* occurs, there is only the background stillness. This moment is when the mind is liberated and no longer influenced by thoughts.

Practicing *samyama* on these three modifications eliminates the distractions of the mind, allowing it to travel beyond the ordinary perception of time. If the same *samyama* is applied to the characteristic, time state, and condition of an object, the purified mind of a yogi can know the events leading to the object's appearance and infer its potential in the future.

EXERCISE:

Look at your face very closely in the mirror. Can you see into your past and future?

Your Past Lives Are Within

3.18 BY *SAMYAMA* ON PAST IMPRESSIONS (*SAMSKARAS*), KNOWLEDGE OF PAST BIRTHS IS GAINED.

Everything that we experience is said to occur due to actions in this life or past lives. The impressions that are stored in memory are inaccessible to the outwardly directed mind. If we practice *samyama* on any of these impressions, we can go deep into the subconscious mind and see the chain of cause and effect that produced them, even if they originated early in childhood.

It is the desire to know and experience that brings about the life cycle. Yogis believe that the soul ends the cycle of reincarnation once these desires are exhausted or overcome. If *samyama* is practiced on the changes in the characteristic, time state, and condition of *samskaras*, you will notice that some of these karmic impressions are working now, some are worked out, and some are waiting to be worked out.

There are cases of yoga masters who have seen visions of their past lives before ultimate liberation. Even in scientific studies, children between the ages of two and six years old have been able to recount stories that were traced back to actual people who died years before.

REFLECTION:

Think about an experience in your past. Is there a logical reason you had that experience? Think back to the causes of your memories and experiences.

Knowing the Mind-Set of Others

3.19 BY *SAMYAMA* ON IDEAS, ONE CAN KNOW THE THOUGHTS OF OTHERS.

It is sometimes possible to know the thoughts of other people by observing their body language, their face, or their voice. You can tell if someone is lying to you if they look uncomfortable or their voice changes. This ability is a common skill that most people can learn.

Yogis who practice concentration, meditation, and absorption on ideas understand their own minds to such an extent that they can actually know the thoughts of other people. By knowing the beliefs, attitudes, and values of someone, you know their mind-set.

Think of a piano teacher who is teaching someone a piece of music. There might be a section of the song that is difficult to play. If the teacher has also worked through that section, they know exactly what is going on in the mind of the student, which helps them be a better teacher.

By the practice of *samyama* on ideas, the yogi's mind becomes like an antenna that can pick up thought waves and transmit them. There are stories of yogis who could visit remote places without physically going anywhere, share teachings with their students in dreams, and travel outside of their bodies to bring back knowledge.

REFLECTION:

Think about the last time you had a conversation with someone. Could you tell when they were exaggerating or appeared to be dishonest?

Predicting Death

3.22 BY *SAMYAMA* ON KARMA (WHICH IS EITHER IN MOTION OR NOT IN MOTION) OR ON WARNING SIGNS, KNOWLEDGE OF ONE'S TIME OF DEATH CAN BE ACQUIRED.

In India and other parts of the world, there are many cases of people who were able to predict the date and time of their own death. It is said that a natural death comes when the soul has exhausted the karmas of its current life and is ready to move on to its next life. For this reason, suicide is not a good choice on the spiritual path.

In the ancient Indian medical system of Ayurveda, various warning signs of death (called *arishtas*) can be noticed from the pulse, voice, smells, and dreams of a person. Death can be delayed by the blessing of holy men or by the use of drugs.

STORY:

I was studying in the ashram of a very powerful yogi. One night he called a student into the room and told her that he was going to leave his body. He repeated some mantras and that was it! The next day, we had a chance to witness his lifeless body, sitting upright in the lotus position. He was buried that same day.

Making Friends, Not Enemies

3.23 BY *SAMYAMA* ON QUALITIES LIKE FRIENDLINESS, COMPASSION, AND HAPPINESS, THE YOGI BECOMES POWERFUL.

Have you noticed that some people look more friendly? Or that when someone enters the room, there is a change in the atmosphere? The real power of a yogi comes from the quality of their life. As a yogi practices concentration, meditation, and absorption on positive qualities, their entire being radiates that quality.

As a yogi masters nonviolence, aggressive animals become docile and calm around them. If they practice friendliness, they can become a friend to everyone. If they focus on happiness, they can transmit happiness to other people.

Your character and reality are both built on the thoughts and feelings on which you focus. So, if you always have negative or violent thoughts, you are more likely to experience negativity and violence.

There is a practice called loving-kindness meditation where you repeat in your mind a phrase like "May all beings live with ease; may all beings be free; may all beings be free from pain." As you practice for several minutes, your inner being is transformed.

REFLECTION:

Think of someone who makes you happy and someone who makes you sad. Who is more powerful and influential?

Harness the Power of the Mind

3.24 BY *SAMYAMA* ON PHYSICAL STRENGTH, THE STRENGTH OF AN ELEPHANT OR OTHERS CAN BE GAINED.

By the power of concentration, meditation, and absorption, yogis can draw into themselves any power or quality found in nature. In *samadhi* (absorption), the self and the object meditated upon become one. If one chooses to focus on the speed of a horse, for example, they can run faster. If the focus is on the fluidity of water, one can dance more gracefully. We can use the power of the mind to help us.

Many yoga *asanas* are named after animals because thinking of the animal increases your focus and gives you that animal's strength. For example, *Bhujangasana* is the Cobra Pose. This back-bending and strengthening pose is more effective if you focus on how easily the cobra can lift its upper body.

One of my teachers told me that for some psychological conditions, like schizophrenia, a mantra for the elephant-headed deity Ganesh is prescribed. Because the elephant is a heavy and strong animal, this mantra creates a grounding feeling and stabilization of the mind for people whose mind is constantly moving.

EXERCISE:

Think about a physical ability or trait that you wish to have. Next, choose an animal or person that excels at that ability. Bring that animal or person to mind when you need strength and inspiration.

Your Real Center

3.34 BY *SAMYAMA* ON THE MYSTIC HEART, KNOWLEDGE OF THE MIND IS ACQUIRED.

When a person says "I," they often touch the center of their chest. Because the heart center is the seat of the ego, it organizes all of our experiences. We are thinking, feeling, and doing beings. The heart chakra is in the center of the subtle body system and is where the physical nature, which is controlled by the lower centers, meets the upper chakras related to higher centers of thought and ability.

Our deepest motivations are based on feelings and not thoughts. Most of the choices we make are because we want to feel something or to avoid negative feelings. Even in the brain, the emotional center is essential for consciousness.

The emotional heart is where we hold attachments and desires. It is also where the qualities of love and compassion are developed. In the process of spiritual unfolding, the experience of expansion and opening occurs in the heart. The result of the highest knowledge and intellectual insight is universal compassion and love for everyone and everything.

EXERCISE:
Spend a few moments feeling your heart center and your emotions. Send yourself pure love and extend this feeling to all of humanity.

Right Use of Power

3.37 POWERS ARE ACCOMPLISHMENTS TO THE OUTWARDLY FOCUSED MIND BUT OBSTACLES TO *SAMADHI.*

There are many people who have extraordinary skills in music who are also blind. Maybe it is because the sense of sight is unused that the sense of hearing is enhanced. In fact, any skill that you want to improve usually requires sacrificing others.

With the various practices of yoga, the mind and body are challenged to their extremes, and many capabilities can arise. For example, if you pay close attention to your emotions and the movements of your mind, it is a lot easier to win arguments against people whose thinking is clouded by their feelings.

The sincere yogi, however, is not interested in using their powers to win debates, become famous, or make money. If a yogi demonstrates their powers, they will only attract more attention and become involved in outward karma, which can create more distractions for the inward-focused mind. Yogic powers, which can naturally arise, should simply encourage more practice. Powers can be useful in the service of others, but one should not allow them to distract from the process of purifying the deeper mind and ego.

REFLECTION:
What kind of capabilities has yoga revealed in your life?

The Lightness of Being

3.39 BY MASTERY OVER THE UPWARD MOVING ENERGY IN THE BODY (*UDANA VAYU*), THE YOGI CAN FLOAT OVER WATER, WALK ON THORNS, AND LEAVE THE BODY AT WILL.

There are five basic directions of movement of subtle life force within the body that control different functions. *Prana vayu* brings energy into the body. *Vyana vayu* distributes energy throughout the body. *Samana vayu* is involved in centralizing and integrating energy. *Apana vayu* moves energy down and outward, and *udana vayu* moves energy upward.

Every yoga *asana* affects these subtle movements of energy within. Even our emotions influence them. As a result, after the practice of yoga, the energies in the body become harmonized and regulated. With mastery of *pranayama*, many powers are gained, including the power to levitate, which has been demonstrated by yogis and saints.

If you have ever had the experience of vomiting, or felt lightness in the body from uplifting positive emotions, you have felt the power of *udana vayu*. This energy is also responsible for keeping the body upright, and advanced yogis use it to exit their body through the crown of the head at the time of death.

EXERCISE:

Straighten your back and raise your hands over your head for two to three minutes. Notice how your mood and enthusiasm change. Use this exercise throughout the day whenever you need a mental boost.

Developing Your Aura

3.40 BY MASTERY OVER THE STABILIZING ENERGY (*SAMANA VAYU*), THE YOGI'S BODY GLOWS.

The naval region is where the fire principle is active. There, the heat of metabolism and digestion, which fuels the body, is controlled by the vital force called *samana vayu*. A basic principle in Ayurvedic medicine is that improper digestion of food is a major cause of illness. If digestion is weak or overwhelmed, the body becomes toxic and inefficient.

Through the practices of fasting, *asana*, *pranayama*, and celibacy, energy is conserved and magnified to such a high level that a yogi's body appears to glow. This glow is an extension of the immune system, which when fully charged can repel diseases and even spread healing energy to others.

When people are nervous, they can feel uneasiness in the belly, confusion, and a lack of hunger. The naval region itself is like a second brain that needs to function well in order to integrate information and feelings.

EXERCISE:

Take a moment and feel your belly from within. Notice what kinds of messages you get from there regarding your feelings and diet.

The Play of the Elements

3.44 BY *SAMYAMA* ON THE GROSS ELEMENTS AND THEIR QUALITIES, SUBTLE NATURE, CORRELATIONS, AND PURPOSE, MASTERY OVER THEM IS GAINED.

The body is a microcosm of the natural world. The elements are mapped in order of density along the spine. The lower part of the body, from the legs to the belly, corresponds to earth, water, and fire. From the chest to the head is air and space. Each element has psychological correlations, too.

In natural healing, the use of opposite qualities helps heal the body and mind. For example, when the body is cold and sluggish from too much earth and water energy, spicy foods with more of the fire element can activate digestion and stimulate the mind to create balance.

When meditation is directed with attention upward, it increases the space element in the mind. Space is also correlated with the perception of sound. A yogi, like a scientist, practices *samyama* on these ideas and realizes that experience refines our relationship to nature. At this point, the yogi is able to ride the rivers of life on the boat of knowledge.

REFLECTION:
Which elements are most active in your life now?

Bodily Perfection

3.45 MASTERY OVER THE FIVE ELEMENTS BRINGS PERFECTION TO THE BODY AND LEADS TO EXTRAORDINARY POWERS, LIKE BEING ABLE TO MAKE ONESELF SMALL AND BECOMING RESISTANT TO OUTSIDE FORCES.

Perfection of the body includes beauty, grace, and strength. When the elements are properly balanced, all of the internal organs work well, digestion is strong, the body is not too hot or too cold, the mind is joyful, and sleep is good. The body works best when it is connected to the rhythms of nature. In its balanced state, you should not even notice it.

A yogi can transform their body in the course of a few days with the use of proper diet, yoga *asana*s, and rest. There are mystic powers related to mastery over the elements, like being able to make the body invisible or as heavy or light as one desires. These powers make you indifferent to outside forces, but they should not be used for personal gain.

STORY:

I heard the story of a yogi who got very close to the floor in order to feed a dog. The people in the room noticed that his entire form appeared to become smaller in order to look the animal in the eyes and not scare it.

Mind Your Senses

3.47 MASTERY OVER THE SENSE ORGANS IS GAINED BY *SAMYAMA* ON THEIR POWER OF PERCEPTION, REAL NATURE, EGOS, QUALITIES, AND PURPOSE.

Each of the five senses presents different knowledge to the soul as it perceives and reports on objects in the outside world. The sense organs help the mind create a mental image of what is outside. When you think of the ears, skin, eyes, tongue, and nose, each seems to have a particular mind of its own. They are not always active at the same time, and some of them have different inclinations or qualities.

A major concept in health and yoga is how much we use our senses and how they control our actions. Some people overuse their hearing and might lose it if they aren't careful while listening to loud music. Overusing the sense of taste can lead to overeating or eating unhealthy foods that lead to obesity or other diseases.

Peace and joy are reestablished when the senses are stabilized by yoga and meditation. We learn to appreciate the senses and start to practice moderation, naturally letting go of addictions and attachments to outside things. After having many enjoyable sensory experiences, we will eventually seek more refined experiences and realizations.

REFLECTION:

What are some senses that you no longer overuse but now use in moderation and with gratitude?

Your True Potential

3.49 BY RECOGNITION OF THE DIFFERENCE BETWEEN THE INTELLECT AND THE SOUL, OMNIPOTENCE (ALL-POWERFULNESS) AND OMNISCIENCE (ALL-KNOWINGNESS) ARE GAINED.

Each of us lives in a world that is defined by what we experience, how we interpret those experiences, and what choices we make. The habits and desires of the mind are what activate the body to move. We might think that the body has a life of its own, but it is also controlled by the nervous system.

The yogi actively takes control of these mechanisms and seeks the highest control center within. When you know how to regulate and control your actions, you become responsible and more impactful in your own reality. That outcome reflects the value of intelligence and discipline. You will gain ultimate independence; no matter what is going on outside, nothing will change within.

The barrier to cross is at the peak of this control when even the intellect and sense of your individual self have to be transcended to realize your true potential. Each person has the same ability to have great thoughts and to achieve great things. The power of the spirit is unlimited; it can help you access any knowledge you need and harness any strength you need to fulfill your worldly or spiritual goals.

REFLECTION:

What areas of your life could use more attention and active engagement?

From Individual to Cosmic

3.50 BY NONATTACHMENT TO EVEN OMNIPOTENCE AND OMNISCIENCE, THE ROOT OF DEFECTS IS DESTROYED AND LIBERATION COMES.

The powerful mental and physical capabilities that come from yoga practice are not the end of the spiritual path. With them, you remain undisturbed by nature and can understand any object or problem—but this is just the beginning.

In Sutra 3.37 (see page 166), Patanjali mentions the problem of misusing the powers on the inner path. Here, he returns to the theme of highest detachment mentioned in Sutra 1.16 (see page 32). The roots of suffering are your attachment to experiences and the belief that you are the temporary mind and body. Revisit Sutra 2.3 (see page 68) and the discussion of *kleshas*.

To know everything and to be all-powerful are the highest superpowers, but they must also be transcended in order to be completely released from suffering and the cycle of rebirth.

The state of liberation is like a feeling of aloneness, but it is also full of the totality of power and knowledge that life has to offer. A yogi who touches this dimension is unlikely to return to pain-causing habits or incorrect notions. Their individual soul has merged with the cosmic spirit.

REFLECTION:

What would you do if you could do anything and know everything?

Spontaneous Action

3.54 ENLIGHTENED KNOWLEDGE THAT SIMULTANEOUSLY COMPREHENDS ALL OBJECTS IS INTUITIVE AND LIBERATING.

Life is a sequence of single moments, and your personal reality is all you really know. When you are identified with the spirit, you are free from ignorance of your true nature. If at the same time you do not care to know or experience more, you are fully liberated. Then your actions become as effortless as brushing your teeth. What knowledge you need will come to you as it is required. Many people live intuitive lives like this.

By staying grounded in the understanding that your higher self is beyond the play of time and nature, you will realize that activity is spontaneously happening without having to think too much about it. In fact, we are already enlightened. We just don't know it.

STORY:

When I teach yoga, I don't use notes or overly prepare for my classes. I know that the students are there to experience what the teacher must embody. I am doing the best I can and am ready to admit when I do not know something. For me, every moment is an opportunity for deepening in this living art and science. There is a grace and timelessness in doing what you love.

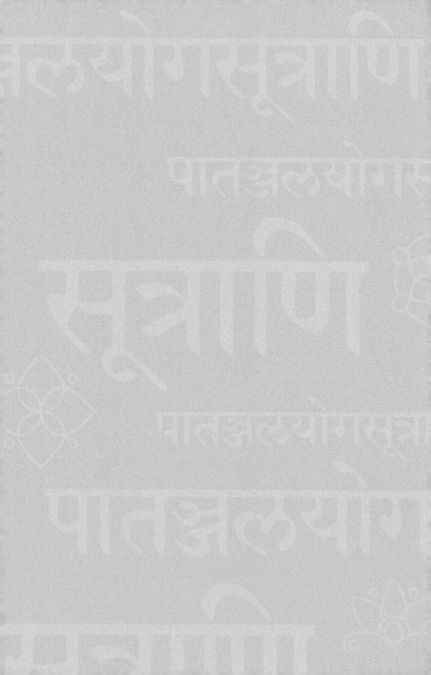

BOOK FOUR

Going Beyond the Mind

The fourth book, known as the Book of
Absolute Independence, explores universal
laws that govern the life of a spiritual being
from birth to final incarnation.

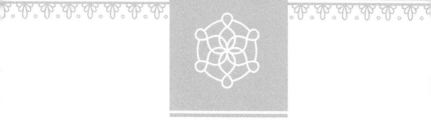

Special Abilities

4.1 SUPERNORMAL POWERS (*SIDDHIS*) COME FROM PAST LIVES, MEDICINAL HERBS, MANTRAS, AUSTERITIES (*TAPAS*), OR *SAMADHI*.

For some seekers, the powers described in Book Three come easily. They may have taken up spiritual practice at an early age, a sign that they have pursued a spiritual path in a previous life. This is why they access supernormal potentials with relative ease.

There are also medicinal formulas called *rasayanas* that are taken to make the body super healthy and allow for powers to awaken. The use of certain other drugs creates altered states of mind, but because of their negative side effects and short-term results, they are not a reliable method for sustained spiritual growth.

Repeating mantras also creates changes in the mind. Some mantras have very specific effects and powers. Austerities, like fasting or holding certain yoga postures for extended periods, can also produce these results. The most reliable and long-lasting effects, however, are by the practices of concentration and meditation leading to absorption (*samadhi*).

My Ayurveda teacher has the ability to diagnose diseases in the mind and body by just looking at the tongue or feeling the pulse of the person who is sick. These very practical abilities require yogic focus and are used to help others.

REFLECTION:

What are some abilities that you easily acquired in this life? How can you use them to help others?

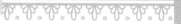

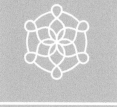

Skill in Action

4.7 THE ACTIONS OF A YOGI ARE NEITHER GOOD NOR BAD, WHEREAS THE ACTIONS OF NON-YOGIS ARE EITHER GOOD, BAD, OR A MIXTURE OF GOOD AND BAD.

Good actions create happiness and do not harm others. Being nonviolent and compassionate always creates more peace around you. Bad actions can be external or internal, like stealing, insulting people, or even planning to hurt others. Most of our actions are a mixture of both. Even when we do something good, there may be a negative effect on another being somewhere.

Also, usually when we do something, we have an expectation of the result. You give someone a gift and get angry if they do not thank you. Maybe you say "I love you" and expect the other person to say it back. This way of thinking creates unpleasant and painful feelings.

A dedicated yogi acts for the sake of acting. They constantly reset their perspective of the present moment while knowing that their inner being is always untouched and independent of the results—demonstrating real skill in action. The yogi keeps the mind fresh by meditation and remains unselfish by seeing themselves as part of the whole creation.

REFLECTION:

Think back to the last time you expected someone to say or do something in reaction to something you said or did for them. Was it fair to have that expectation of them? Now, try thinking about doing something without any expectation. How would this change your feelings during and after the activity?

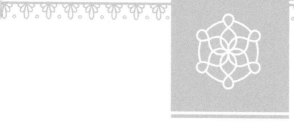

Everything Has a Cause and Effect

4.8 THESE THREE KINDS OF ACTIONS (GOOD, BAD, AND MIXED) CREATE SUBCONSCIOUS IMPRESSIONS, HABITS, AND DESIRES THAT MANIFEST, WHEN CONDITIONS ARE FAVORABLE, IN FUTURE KARMA.

When you treat someone unkindly, there is a response inside of you. Maybe you get a feeling of superiority or strength. This feeling feeds the ego, so you will most likely do it again. Even good actions, like yoga practice, create subconscious impressions that will cause you to practice more.

The theory of karma states that everything has a cause and effect. Even the family in which you are born, your life span, your abilities, and your personality are the results of actions in previous lives. This life and future lives exist for you to experience the results of actions and exhaust these karmic seeds, tendencies, and desires.

By practicing yoga, you can stop accumulating negative impressions (*samskaras*). You can stop seeking environments and opportunities to repeat bad actions. Yogis accept suffering as a source of learning and purification for past karmas. Through practice, they also actively and patiently allow negative subconscious impressions to dissolve and resolve themselves.

REFLECTION:

Do you notice patterns in your behavior that you wish to change? How can you protect yourself from environments that cause you to repeat those actions?

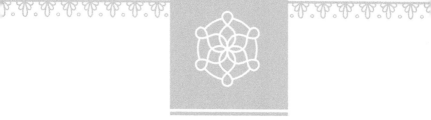

Karma University

4.11 KARMIC TENDENCIES EXIST DUE TO THE RELATIONSHIP OF CAUSE AND EFFECT AND THE ASSOCIATION OF THE MIND WITH OBJECTS. WHEN IGNORANCE (THE CAUSE OF SELFISH ACTIONS), MEMORY (THE EFFECT OF ACTIONS), AND THE MIND'S ASSOCIATION WITH NATURE DISAPPEAR, SO DO IMPRESSIONS AND DESIRES.

Karmic tendencies are rooted in the senses and the mind, which records memories. Objects in the outside world support the continuation of these memories and desires. We cannot remove the objects of the world or the mind. We have to change our perspective. When we practice meditation, changing our perspective is exactly what we are doing.

The cause of our binding actions begins with the ignorance of not knowing our real nature. We are spiritual beings and our life's purpose is to realize this truth. Nature has a way of pulling us in and then teaching us that we should not get attached to her.

There is no need to fight our desires or attachments. Slowly, they will fall away if we pay attention and learn. The ultimate effect of karma is the cycle of rebirth; we stay in the university of life until we are ready to graduate.

REFLECTION:

As you learn about spiritual life and perspectives, how have your actions, desires, and the impressions you consume changed?

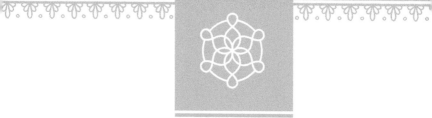

Spiritual Quantum Physics

4.14 THE REALITY OF THINGS IS DUE TO COMBINATIONS OF THE BASIC QUALITIES OF NATURE (*GUNAS*).

Imagine that your entire being is recreated every moment. The three basic forces of nature—lightness (*sattva*), movement (*rajas*), and stability (*tamas*)—interact with each other to create the ego, mind, senses, and all of the elements of the body. When one is more active, the others are less active or act as support.

The mind is a product of the *sattva guna*. Its original nature is pure and full of knowledge, but if there is overactivity or laziness, then it loses its naturally meditative state. When *rajas* is strongest, the organs of action (such as feet, hands, and the mouth) are generated. The elements of the body are a product of *tamas*.

When there is perfect balance between these three forces, nothing is created or experienced; what remains is the raw potential of nature and the spirit (both of which never change). In one form of meditation, you mentally trace the process of creation in reverse order. In the liberated state—due to the exhaustion of karma—the *gunas* no longer create a body.

REFLECTION:

We live in a world of infinite possibilities. Science tells us that quantum-scale objects exist as either particles or waves. This nonintuitive reality reflects the spiritual world view as well.

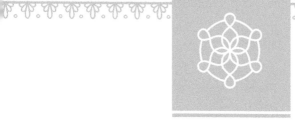

Perceptions Differ

4.15 DUE TO DIFFERENCES IN VARIOUS MINDS, THE SAME OBJECT IS PERCEIVED DIFFERENTLY.

How many different ways do people experience a painting, food, or music? In the process of perceiving objects of the world, each person brings their own perspective and judgments. The experiences we have and the actions that we take alter the *gunas* (qualities) of the mind. In turn, changes in the *gunas* affect how we take in impressions and our response.

How we manage our mental energy and the biases and projections that we impose on perception are completely our own. Reality is not constructed for the benefit of just one person; each of us has our own karmic path to live out. In fact, perception and reactions are karma!

STORY:

I always tell yoga trainees that they should not wear clothing with logos or words on them. They cannot know what kind of reaction it will create in the students. Maybe one of the students doesn't like that band or has a negative association with that team. A yoga teacher's job is to help students calm and clarify their minds. Only then can karmic impressions be released.

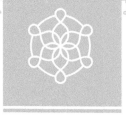

Coloring the Mind

4.17 A THING IS KNOWN OR UNKNOWN BY THE MIND DEPENDING ON WHETHER IT IS NOTICED BY THE MIND.

Your interests determine what the mind notices—including sensory perceptions and concepts. The mind is like a canvas that gets painted by objects. The more intently you focus on something, the deeper the color of the paint and the more knowledge you gain from the object. For example, when you study for an exam, often you have to concentrate on the same concept many times before you understand or are able to memorize it.

Sometimes a traumatic event can create a painful memory for someone. Then they may overreact to situations because of impressions in the subconscious mind. This irrational behavior can create problems in life and relationships. Until you shed the light of awareness on that experience, feelings and thoughts cannot be properly processed. A mind that is clear and fresh absorbs what it chooses and reflects the true reality of each moment.

STORY:

In high school, I started to take the bus. After regularly using public transportation, I began to notice buses all around town. I never noticed them before that time.

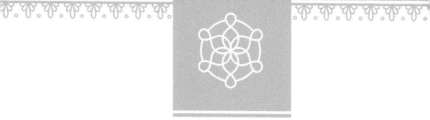

The Mind Cannot Multitask

4.20 THE MIND CANNOT PERCEIVE
BOTH THE SOUL AND OBJECTS AT THE
SAME TIME.

The mind is energized by the soul (or spirit) to receive and process information about the environment and the body. It perceives objects and makes a copy to present to the soul for its enjoyment and liberation. When the mind is busy with these processes, it cannot at the same time be aware of the soul that is in the background.

The soul is always aware of the changes that are happening in the mind. Sadly, the wisdom that arises from reflecting on the soul is missed as we fight to survive, avoid dangers, and seek sensory pleasures.

When we go to sleep, there is some feedback from the soul. People often wake up realizing the answer to a problem because the mind took time off from worrying about the problem while it rested. Meditation is like sleep. When the mind is made calm and clear, it can turn within to perceive the soul. Then you realize your true nature and your perspective, motivations, and actions change.

REFLECTION:

Have you ever watched yourself doing more than one thing at a time? Has multitasking served you in accomplishing your goals?

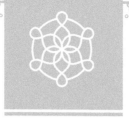

Desires Cause Rebirth

4.24 THOUGH HAVING COUNTLESS DESIRES, THE MIND EXISTS FOR THE SAKE OF THE SOUL BECAUSE IT CAN ACT ONLY IN ASSOCIATION WITH THE SOUL.

When you are able to say "I am happy" or "I am sad," it proves that there is an awareness within you that is noticing these changes. The changes are happening by momentary combinations of the qualities of nature (*gunas*) in the mind. The mind does not act for itself. The states of the mind are presented to the soul for its enjoyment and ultimately so that the mind can be transcended in liberation.

The mind takes on the goals of the soul. Every desire and action that you have has at its root some seeking of experience by the soul. This seeking is a beautiful thing, but actually it's a problem that must be overcome in order to liberate the soul from the cycle of rebirth. Whenever you are reborn in a human form due to unresolved desires, the mind undergoes bondage, ignorance, and suffering.

In meditation, it is possible to access the soul that is actually never suffering. In those moments when you are not identified with the mind, body, and ego, you experience the nature of the soul and are freed from psychological suffering. That experience is similar to liberation.

EXERCISE:
Write down all of the experiences you really want to have in this life.

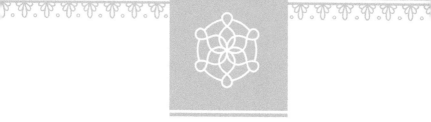

Who Am I?

4.25 FOR THOSE WHO KNOW THE DISTINCTION BETWEEN THE MIND AND THE SOUL, QUESTIONS REGARDING THE NATURE OF THE SOUL COME TO AN END.

The expression "I think, therefore I am" is true but not because you exist when you think. It's true because the "I am" ego sense is created when you think. You do not need to think in order to exist! Existence and awareness are the nature of the soul. The soul that each of us has is part of the cosmic soul that is undying.

Because the mind and the soul are very closely connected to each other, you believe that they are the same. There is a meditation practice where you repeat the question "Who am I?" silently in your mind. This questioning leads you to the experience of the soul, which is the origin of the mind and all thoughts.

When we start on the inner path, people ask questions: "What is the purpose of life?" "What happens after death?" "Who am I?" As we progress on the path of self-awareness, these questions no longer haunt us. We get connected to the power of the soul and experience intuitive inner guidance and peace. Then, we are naturally aware of the distinction between the soul and the egoistic mind, and we move toward liberation.

EXERCISE:
The next time you feel sad or hungry, do not say "I am sad" or "I am hungry." Say "My mind is sad" or "My body is hungry" instead. Notice how this simple turn of phrase changes your mind-set.

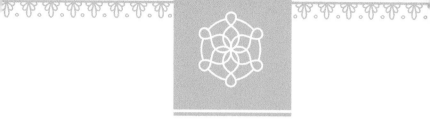

Keep Practicing

4.27 DURING BREAKS IN ENLIGHTENED KNOWLEDGE, OTHER THOUGHTS ARISE DUE TO REMAINING PAST IMPRESSIONS.

Even advanced yogis who have practiced constantly experience the return of past impressions and habits if they lose their concentration. These attachments and impressions might come from past lives or from experiences before they started practicing yoga.

Usually, because their practice is so strong, these thoughts are immediately released. However, there are examples of yogis who achieved great things and then fell back into selfishness, egoism, and attachment. Although they can point you in the right direction and remove darkness from within you, it is best not to blindly glorify any teacher.

Seeking the highest wisdom brings knowledge and power, which can be abused. Anyone who is still in a body has karma left to exhaust. Perfection on the human level is practically unattainable. When someone eats or goes to the bathroom, there must be identification at some level with the body.

REFLECTION:
Don't worry about being on the right path. If you are reading this book with real interest, you are on the right track. Any effort to practice, study, and understand yoga is a step in the right direction.

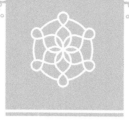

Beyond Knowledge and Power

4.29 WHEN THERE IS NO INTEREST EVEN IN THE HIGHEST STATES DUE TO CONSTANT ENLIGHTENED KNOWLEDGE, THE *SAMADHI* CALLED *DHARMAMEGHA* (THE CLOUD OF TRUTH) COMES.

Eventually, the realization of the distinction between the mind and the soul (discriminative discernment) becomes permanent. The effort to realize the true self, which is beyond the mind and body, somehow causes the secrets of the universe and the powers of nature to be revealed to the dedicated yogi.

Supernormal knowledge and power come through repeated experiences of *samadhi* (meditative absorption). Yogis who realize that abusing these powers brings pain in the changing world develop supreme nonattachment to them. They also develop nonattachment to enlightened knowledge and omniscience. Even though their effort up to this point was toward liberation, it is when even that effort is released that full liberation actually begins.

Because there is nothing left to know, the mind is no longer interested in or pulled toward the outside world. These yogis experience a drowsy trance state full of spontaneous knowledge and bliss. They have no interest or desires left and completely surrender their identity to the greater universe. They might continue to act in the world but are completely unattached.

STORY:

When I have met advanced yogis, I felt like they could see right through me. In their presence, my mind becomes still and reflects their love and compassion.

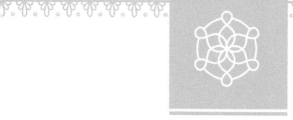

Ultimate Truth

4.34 PERFECT INDEPENDENCE IS REALIZED WHEN, HAVING PROVIDED EXPERIENCE AND LIBERATION FOR THE SOUL, THE QUALITIES (*GUNAS*) ARE REABSORBED BACK INTO NATURE AND THE POWER OF THE SOUL IS ESTABLISHED IN ITSELF.

If you have no more desires, have no more lessons to learn, have no interest to know anything more, have no linear experience of time, have no sense of a separate self or mind, and feel only peace and independence, you have attained liberation. A person in such a condition does not experience rebirth when they die. They are established in truth always and have no more afflictions and ignorance regarding the nature of spiritual reality.

Every one of us is on the same journey. If any concepts in this book ring true to your experience, know that the rest will also be revealed in time. Life is not a prison but a majestic story in which we are all being led to a glorious ending of realization. It will happen for both you and me.

Make an effort to train your mind and body. Learn from your experiences and from others. Stay optimistic and become a portal for service, peace, and understanding. The love and compassion that you embody and express are the light of ultimate truth.

REFLECTION:

One more time, make a connection to your universal spirit. It has been and always will be with you.

RESOURCES

Raja Yoga by Swami Sivananda
A succinct and classical commentary by a renowned yoga master. I also recommend the works of Master Sivananda's disciples: Swami Satchidananda, Swami Satyananda, and Swami Venkatesananda.

The Science of Yoga by I.K. Taimni
An opinionated and thorough interpretation for advanced study.

Self Comes to Mind by Antonio Damasio
An excellent book for a modern scientific perspective on consciousness as well as evolutionary biology.

Yoga and Ayurveda by Dr. David Frawley
An excellent book on yoga philosophy and practices as well as subtle principles involved in healing the mind and body.

Yoga Philosophy of Patanjali by Swami Hariharananda Aranya
The best resource for serious students who want a traditional approach.

Yoga Sutras of Patanjali by Baba Hari Dass
A series of study guides for traditional and comprehensive commentaries on the sutras, especially good for understanding books 3 and 4.

The Yoga Sutras of Patanjali by Edwin F. Bryant
A scholarly resource on the sutras full of cross-references to other traditional commentaries.

"Yoga Sutras of Patanjali: The 196 Sutras" by Swami Jnaneshvara Bharati
https://www.swamij.com/yoga-sutras-list.htm
A useful online resource with many illustrations and commentaries even beyond the sutras.

ACKNOWLEDGMENTS

I am eternally grateful to my mother, who was my first yoga teacher; my father, who taught me how to be a man; and my brother, who deeply influenced my interest in science and the arts. Their examples, love, and support have been my anchor.

Without my teachers and mentors I would not have had the experience or confidence to write such a book. I am especially grateful to my dear friend Reetesh Dwevedi, who invited me into his home and taught me the way of devotion (Bhakti Yoga).

Thank you to my editor Rochelle Torke for her excellent suggestions and the team at Callisto Media for developing the concept and design for this book.

Any of my glimpses into the truth would not have been possible without the inspired works of dedicated practitioners and scholars on whose shoulders we all stand.

ABOUT THE AUTHOR

Ram Bhakt studied neurobiology and music in college. His interests in science, psychology, philosophy, and athletics naturally led him to dive deeply into the yogic practices and tradition. He lived and studied the teachings of Swami Satchidananda at Yogaville Ashram for two years. While there, he was introduced to Ayurvedic medicine and Vedanta by Dr. David Frawley.

Ram's Raja Yoga studies led him to Swami Janakananda, who initiated him into Kriya Yoga. He continues to study with various teachers from all over the world and has shared yoga with children, teens, adults, and seniors. As the founder of Long Beach School of Yoga, he has trained 100-plus teachers and witnessed the impact of yoga on the lives of countless others.